Curriculum Process in Nursing: A Guide to Curriculum Development

Gertrude Torres, Ed. D.
Professor of Nursing
Division of Nursing
D'Youville College
Buffalo, N.Y.

Marjorie Stanton, Ed. D.
Chairperson
Division of Nursing
D'Youville College
Buffalo, N.Y.

PRENTICE-HALL, INC., Englewood Cliffs, New Jersey 07632

Library of Congress Cataloging in Publication Data

Torres, Gertrude.
  Curriculum process in nursing.

  Bibliography: p.
  Includes index.
  1. Nursing–Study and teaching. 2. Curriculum
planning. I. Stanton, Marjorie. II. Title.
[DNLM: 1. Education, Nursing. 2. Curriculum. WY 18
T693n]
RT71.T67   610.73'07'11   81-4636
ISBN 0-13-196261-2   AACR2

Editorial production and supervision by Maria McKinnon
Interior design by Maria McKinnon
Cover design by George Alon Jaediker
Manufacturing buyer: John Hall

PRENTICE-HALL INTERNATIONAL, INC., *London*
PRENTICE-HALL OF AUSTRALIA PTY. LIMITED, *Sydney*
PRENTICE-HALL OF CANADA, LTD., *Toronto*
PRENTICE-HALL OF INDIA PRIVATE LIMITED, *New Delhi*
PRENTICE-HALL OF JAPAN, INC., *Tokyo*
PRENTICE-HALL OF SOUTHEAST ASIA PTE. LTD., *Singapore*
WHITEHALL BOOKS LIMITED, *Wellington, New Zealand*

This book is dedicated to those faculty, graduate students, and under-graduate students in nursing who worked with us, shared their ideas, challenged our thinking, and who above all, remain painfully steadfast and true to the ideals of integrity and autonomy of nursing education.

Contents

Preface

All faculty members in nursing, regardless of the setting, will be involved in the planning, development, and implementation of a curriculum at some point in their professional lives.

Each of us has spent considerable time over the years in curriculum consultation and have found that while faculty may have knowledge about curriculum theory, it is fragmented and often not useful in the actual practice of designing and implementing a curriculum. Many of these faculty members have urged us to write a book that could be helpful in the day-to-day development of a curriculum.

It is assumed that readers of this book will have reviewed the abounding literature related to curriculum theory. This book is not intended to be used in isolation. Its goal is to provide practical ideas about how to use the curriculum process to develop, implement, and evaluate a curriculum in nursing. Approaches to curriculum development are dynamic, changing, and responsive to unique circumstances. Our thinking and approaches have changed and emerged, as readers familiar with our previous writing will see. For example, this text presents an approach that does not include a conceptual framework, but uses rather a theoretical framework.

There are essentially four areas of focus. The introduction, Chapter 1, gives an overview of the subject and identifies forces that impact on curriculum process. Chapters 2 through 5 focus on the four stages of the curriculum process: the directive stage, the formative stage, the functional stage, and the evaluative stage. Chapter 6 provides a sample curriculum to assist the reader's understanding of the curriculum process. Chapter 7, the last chapter, focuses on the development of curricula to accommodate the transfer student, particularly the registered nurse student. At the conclusion of the book, a glossary of terms and a reference list is included. Each area builds on the other so that it is essential to read the text in its presented sequence. It is our hope that the guidelines presented in this book will stimulate the faculty member or student to continually find and create better ways to prepare the future generation of nurses.

Many of our ideas and writings have been influenced by the criticism and challenging views of our peers, graduate students, and other experts in the area of curriculum development from whom we continue to learn.

Special appreciation is expressed to Helen Yura, Ph.D., for her review of the manuscript, support of our efforts, and involvement with the early development of the conceptual framework for nursing education.

Gertrude Torres

Dayton, Ohio   Marjorie Stanton

Introduction

Curriculum development in nursing consumes much time and energy on the part of faculty. Whether it occurs within the framework of a two- or four-year educational institution or a staff development program in an agency, the resources that are used to develop the curriculum package are expensive. Every effort needs to be made so that the development of quality education can take place in the most economical and least stressful manner. This means using resources effectively. One of the most significant resources is a faculty that is wise and understanding in the use of the curriculum process.

Faculty Responsibility

The faculty of any given program or department is responsible for the development and implementation of the curriculum. However, the ability of individual faculty members to engage in curriculum development or in fact to teach varies widely in and among nursing programs. It is understood that faculty members in nursing must have graduate preparation in nursing as a discipline, preferably at the doctoral level. This background is the impetus for providing students of professional nursing with the knowledge, skills, and attitudes necessary to practice nursing. While knowledge of the discipline is unquestioned, it is equally important that the faculty be able to organize and implement a curriculum which makes sense and can be evaluated.

Many college or university faculties, whatever the discipline, have little or no educational background in curriculum and teaching. Therefore, it becomes necessary for them to avail themselves of the resources available in the literature and in the academic community.

It may be necessary for a total faculty or selected faculty members to participate in continuing education programs in the curriculum process. This is suggested prior to any major curriculum change. It is also suggested from time to time, either as new faculty members are employed or to update faculty members. This could take many forms such as a review of the literature or of attending conferences and workshops related to the approach to the curriculum that is being developed. Another effective method which is infrequently used is to share the expertise within a faculty to provide in-service programs. There is usually a wealth of knowledge and experience within a faculty group that can be used to implement a modified or changed curriculum.

Consultants may be helpful if they are selected carefully in terms of their specific area of expertise and the specific needs of the faculty. It should be remembered that consultants provide input which may or may not be useful to the faculty. They assist the faculty but they should not direct the faculty. In using any consultant, faculty members should be clear as to whether they need assistance in process and/or content. Process relates to the faculty's need to understand the dynamics of curriculum development and the curriculum process. Content relates to the knowledge about curriculum and nursing that is essential to support the process. For example, the components of a philosophy and the theoretical knowledge related to health and nursing are *content* while the approach to the utilization of that knowledge to develop a philosophy is *process*. Whatever form of support is provided to the faculty, it should be recognized that curriculum development is a learning experience in and of itself.

In order to engage in curriculum development as an ongoing process, a commitment is needed on the part of the nursing administration, the faculty, and students. Without this commitment time and energy are wasted. The curriculum process becomes an academic exercise instead of a useful and productive tool. It is essential that both administration and faculty of the nursing program are committed to the activity. If either is not, implementation is almost impossible. The administration provides the resources, especially in terms of the quality and quantity of the faculty and it should provide leadership in the role of a catalyst. The faculty offers its expertise both in the areas of practice and education and it has the major role in the total development and maintenance of any program. It also has the responsibility of implementing the curriculum. If students do not know their role in the process, they become frustrated. Their major role is to provide the input which assists in ongoing evaluation. Failure is inevitable unless everyone involved accepts responsibility and views such an activity as a priority.

Organizational Structure

Key to the development of a curriculum is an organizational structure that is conducive to the task. The organizational structure must be flexible so that it can be modified as the curriculum approach changes. Organizational structures once set are almost impossible to change since they reflect the concept of territoriality. Programs oriented to the medical model specialities such as medical–surgical and psychiatric nursing have traditionally supported medical model oriented curricula and departments. If during the development of a revised curriculum a different model evolves, a reorganization of the educational unit may be necessary to ensure success. Generally speaking, the organizational structure of a unit works best if it relates to the philosophical position of the faculty. A philosophy which speaks strongly to the developmental needs of people might very well have departments of nursing of infants and children, nursing of adolescents, nursing of adults, and nursing of the elderly. A philosophy emphasizing the health–illness continuum might consider departments of health nursing, chronic and long-term illness nursing, and acute illness nursing. The structure of the unit helps to support the developed curriculum and it also provides a mechanism to focus research efforts and to recruit and retain qualified faculty. Thus, it must be recognized that changes in curriculum may have a strong impact on the structure of the existing program.

The structure must clearly differentiate administrative decisions from those made by the faculty and students within an educational unit. For example, the faculty is responsible for the planning, development, and implementation of the curriculum. However, these activities take place in the context of administrative planning and decision making relative to available financial and other resources. For faculty to plan and develop a nursing program that relies heavily on an auto-tutorial lab when there is no budgetary support to provide an autotutorial lab is a sheer waste of time. Faculty decision making also takes into consideration the characteristics of the students. Planning a largely autotutorial program for students who have had little or no experience in independent learning may also be fruitless if students cannot or will not participate.

The role and function of any committee also needs to be established in terms of who makes final decisions. Unless there is clarity, frustration and conflict will evolve. This is especially important in terms of curriculum decisions since confusion in the decision-making process will dramatically impede the development of any curriculum. A committee structure that allows for the faculty to function as a curriculum committee of the whole has many advantages. Since all faculty members are involved in the implementation of the curriculum, it is essential that they be kept informed and that they provide input on an ongoing basis. This does not negate the need for ad hoc groups to accomplish specific tasks. Ad hoc committees are different from subcommittees which have the total responsibility of developing the curriculum and reporting back to the faculty for approval. All too often a small group of faculty members initially develops a curriculum or is assigned to do so within an ongoing program during the summer or on released time. Rarely is this an effective mechanism since communications break down and the commitments to the developed curriculum are substantially lessened. The potential for success in terms of curriculum implementation is directly related to the degree of participation on the part of the total faculty. *The greater the amount of participation of the faculty, the greater the degree of success.*

The committee structure must allow not only for day-to-day changes but also for changes in the future. Resources in terms of time and energy may have to be shifted to or from other committees. A total analysis of the organizational structure which supports curriculum change will have to be made. There is probably no better way to resist change than to have committees charged with unrealistic goals and without adequate resources and support.

Timetable

One of the most useful tools in achieving any goal is the development of a realistic timetable that will guide the activities of a group. A written timetable places the activity in the context of its priority and the group's commitment to the goal. Significant to the development of a timetable is whether the potential curriculum changes will impact on the present student group, and if so, at what point. For example, if there are to be changes in the general education or supporting courses, implementation will need to start with incoming students or second-year students. If there are changes in the clinical nursing courses at the junior level, the faculty may decide to revise such prerequisite courses during the year prior to implementation. Thus, the extent of the change must be assessed during the initial stages of curriculum development.

A timetable should include the period of time each component of the curriculum process will be given for development. This period of time is based on the frequency of the meetings. Curriculum development need not be a slow process, but it cannot be effective if intensive crisis-oriented approaches are used. The most productive approach is one that provides regular weekly meetings at which faculty members can assess the results of the decisions step-by-step and can plan for the next activity through studying and creating new ideas. It takes approximately one calendar year to develop or make major changes in a curriculum if there are enough qualified faculty members who have the expertise to do so or who seek assistance and meet on a regularly scheduled basis. Implementation of the curriculum takes longer because it involves the total length of the program. It is not practical to have the faculty spend an intensive period of time on any one component or on developing or revising an entire curriculum because it would tend to be nonproductive in terms of time and energy. There would not be enough time between curriculum decisions for the faculty to assess the significance of the decisions, especially in terms of their impact on the future.

Forces Impacting
on Curriculum Development

There are many forces that will have an impact on the development and implementation of the curriculum in a nursing program. These need to be taken into account as the faculty, with the support and leadership of the nursing program administration, becomes involved with the curriculum process.

The nature and characteristics of the parent institution

that houses the nursing program give direction to and set limits for any department or program within it. Knowing the history of the institution and its mission, purposes, and goals is extremely important and helpful to the faculty of a particular academic unit when planning curricula. A two-year community college, a university, and a liberal arts college have, by nature, very different missions and each provides a different environment for the development of a curriculum in nursing. A natural time limit is imposed by the structure of the institution which sets limits for the nursing program. A state-supported college or university differs from a private college or university not only in the area of financial support but also in purpose. A church-related institution differs from a secular institution. A commuter campus poses different considerations from a dormitory campus where the majority of students are more available and perhaps are a more captive audience. The age of the institution or how long it has been in existence not only influences its financial status but also its traditions, both of which are important considerations in curriculum development.

A parent institution which includes a medical center or health sciences center often provides an environment which is *not* without stress for the development of a nursing curriculum. An administrative structure of a parent institution which does not provide for the autonomy and integrity of all of its academic programs, including nursing, is a constant drain on the energy of the institution as a whole and the department or program specifically.

The characteristics of the students enrolled in the nursing program also have an impact on curriculum planning. The age, cultural background, educational background, family and work responsibilities, expectations, knowledge and feelings about nursing, and the interest and maturation of students are some of the factors that will have an influence on curriculum development. It would be foolish and useless to develop a curriculum package that cannot be implemented for part-time study on a commuter campus where the median age of the nursing student is 28 and where 80 percent of the students work full time to support themselves and their families.

The quantity and quality of the faculty available to the nursing program are vital factors in curriculum development and/or revision. A qualified faculty sufficient in number to plan, develop, and implement a curriculum takes top priority. Many a program has faltered because one qualified person has planned and developed a program which could not be implemented by an unprepared faculty.

Trends

Faculty members must also concern themselves with the changes that will occur in the health care system within the next decade. Of what value is it to develop a curriculum in nursing when most of the learning experiences take place in hospitals or acute care settings if the nature of the health care system is leaning toward preventive and home care. We owe it to students to provide them with knowledge and skills that will prepare them to function in the future, since they will be practicing in the future. Their graduation date is in the future. We also need to teach students how to learn so that they will continue to learn long after they leave the safe and structured environment of the college or university.

The increasing emphasis on the moral and ethical issues involved in providing health care in our technological society will require the concerted efforts of administration, faculty, students, and consumers if we are to keep the nursing profession humanistic in nature. This will not be easy in an era that will be stressing conservation of energy, cutting costs and services, and increased productivity which may mean quantity rather than quality.

Political and legislative activities relating to national health insurance, control of practice, health policies, and the Equal Rights Amendment may have a profound effect on the learning needs of students. If administrators, faculty, and students keep well informed and involved with these activities and plan and project accordingly, they will help to reduce reaction and produce positive action.

Change

Since curriculum development and the use of the curriculum process are always involved with an element of change, the phenomenon of change must be accepted. Deliberate, planned change is much less stressful and time consuming than sudden and unplanned change. Planned change is purposeful, rewarding, and directional. Unplanned or sudden change leads to a patchwork effect. There is a constant flow of energy used in adding on, filling in, patching up—making do without any way of making sure about what is actually happening. The result is a patchwork quilt type curriculum with little or no relationship between and among the stages of the curriculum process.

Summary

Curriculum development does not take place in a vacuum. It takes place in the context of the parent institution which influences, gives direction to, and sets limits for the development of any curriculum within the academic unit. It takes place within the context of the larger community or society which also has an impact on curriculum development. In fact, a review of curricula during any period of time in history reflects to some extent what was considered important by society at the time. It should also give some idea of what was expected to be important at some future time in history. The point here is that the faculty must use the process in the exciting and stimulating challenge of developing a curriculum using the curriculum process in the context of the college or university, the larger community or society, and the profession.

1

Curriculum
Development:
A Process

The development of curricula in nursing programs has been given a great deal of attention in recent years. No faculty member is immune from participation. It seems reasonable and useful then to use a process of curriculum development that makes sense, can be understood, and can be used by the faculty in a variety of programs. The use of the same curriculum process in developing a curriculum for a particular program does not produce the same curricular design for each program, just as the use of the research process does not produce the same research study. What it does do is ensure that the curriculum design for a particular program makes sense and reflects the faculty's beliefs and ideas. Use of the curriculum process provides faculty members with a framework for organizing their ideas and a method for validating their actions.

Nursing has become increasingly "process" directed in the last two decades. This emphasis reflects a growing sophistication and interest in organizing intellectual skills, both in education and in practice. No longer can nursing be content, nor should it be, with simplistic approaches to narrow concerns which do not guide its practitioners into future actions. The educator focuses on the curriculum process to guide learning experiences, the researcher on the research process to find new knowledge, and the practitioner on the nursing process to effect nursing care.

Process

The word process is frequently used and seldom defined, leaving the reader or listener unclear or confused about its meaning. A process involves a series of progressive stages in which interdependent activities have some purpose. A process is systematic, logical, dynamic, and spiraled. It is systematic in nature because it involves an ordered and methodical combination and sequencing of parts into a unitary whole. It is logical because it reflects a continuous and connected series of reasonable stages and steps. As it evolves, it is dynamic yet it suggests a perpetual and long-term commitment. It has a spiral effect because it allows for reassessment and change.

Curriculum Process

Involved in the development of a curriculum is the whole meaning of process. Thus, the curriculum process must reflect all characteristics of a process. It involves a systematic approach to the development of the organized areas of learning and their related aspects. Essential components of the curriculum must evolve in an organized manner and reflect total faculty involvement. Each faculty member must understand and support the essence of a particular curriculum approach so that neither the faculty nor the learners are confused. The curriculum process has the quality of giving direction to the educational program. The curriculum process is logical, moving successfully from one step to the next, showing connections and relationships one to the other. It seems reasonable and makes sense. It is sequential in its approach so that the faculty can use it to identify appropriate actions. It is dynamic in nature in that it is constantly and continuously evolving while providing a sound foundation. There is constant effort to improve the curriculum as both qualitative and quantitative data are gathered. This approach creates a spiraling effect in its forward movement. The spiraling effect of the curriculum process suggests the notion of continuous reassessment and reevaluation.

The curriculum process involves four didactic stages:

1. directive stage

2. formative stage

3. functional stage

4. evaluative stage

Table 1.1 outlines these four stages of the curriculum process. Each stage brings out the significance and purpose of its components. In the early stage of the process it is possible to make revisions, even to moving back and forth from earlier to later stages, but revisions must be made with the awareness that they will affect sequential stages which, in turn, may require other modifications. This supports the belief that each stage closely interacts with and supports the other. The curriculum process can be utilized in either the development of a new curriculum or in the adjustment, revision, modification, or change of an existing one. No curriculum decisions should be made without reviewing the total curriculum. Effectively developed curricula have been rendered useless by frequent piecemeal revisions that have resulted in little interrelationship between and among their parts.

Every effort must be made to develop a common frame of reference so that each stage of the process can be successfully undertaken. As new members join the faculty, a carefully planned sharing of information with them by those who have been longer in the program is essential. This may temporarily slow the process, but in the long run such sharing will prove to be fruitful.

Table 1.1

Stages of the Curriculum Process

STAGE
Directive Gives guidance and authority to the entire curriculum Components: 1. Philosophy 2. Glossary of Terms 3. Characteristics of the Graduate 4. Theoretical Framework
Formative Utilizes the broad, generalized concepts to identify specifics Components: 1. Curriculum Design and Requirements 2. Level and Course Objectives 3. Content Map
Functional Represents the activities affecting the operational component of the curriculum Components: 1. Approaches to Content 2. Teaching Methodology and Learning Experiences 3. Validation of Learning
Evaluative Involves comprehensive, formative, and summative curriculum evaluation Components: 1. Input 2. Throughput 3. Output

Directive Stage

The directive stage of the curriculum process has four components:

1. the philosophy

2. the glossary of terms

3. the characteristics of the graduate

4. the theoretical framework

The directive stage provides the foundation for the development of all subsequent stages and it gives direction to the total curriculum. It is the bulwark of curriculum development. It is in the directive stage that beliefs, theories, concepts, and knowledge are identified; the directive stage is an intellectual activity. A deliberate effort is made to gather sufficient information to make decisions and to give direction to subsequent stages of the curriculum process. The effort, depth, and accuracy given to this stage will significantly affect the total process. Insufficient or inaccurate searches of literature and data gathering lead to poorly developed and inaccurate conclusions and decisions. It should be recognized at this point that the process may be terminated if there is insufficient support for faculty involvement or if there are insufficient resources, especially an adequate number of qualified faculty members. Priorities need to be set since it is not humanly possible to gather data endlessly and it is not humanly possible to attain perfection in this area. There must come a point at which appropriate and adequate factual information is such that the faculty can move in the process. At this stage a step-by-step timetable is helpful for indicating in some detail how much time will be spent on each component. The timetable aids the faculty in gauging its commitment to the program and it provides an incentive to progress. The connections between all components must be clear and obvious to everyone involved in the project. Agreement on priorities and the use of terms must be arrived at in order to make the curriculum operative. Clarity of meaning will thus dispose of ambiguities and misinterpretations.

The development of a philosophy and a glossary of terms to give the philosophy clarity bestow a "categorical imperative" upon the whole curriculum process by setting the course of action which guides the faculty. A faculty engaged in developing a philosophy experiences a realization that, in the end, many beliefs have a common core of agreement. Once the philosophy and the glossary of terms have been agreed upon, the characteristics of the graduate and the theoretical framework may be developed simultaneously since they incorporate the beliefs expressed into theories and concepts and broad objectives.

Since the first stage of the curriculum process requires a great deal of decision making, it may use up a great deal of faculty time and energy. Because concepts and theories may seem abstract and poorly defined, they will at first cause confusion and doubt as to their real purpose. To the faculty members who tend to be more functional in their activities, theorizing appears to serve little purpose. The emphasis of the directive stage accents broadly conceived generalizations and few specifics or details to apply to the real world of everyday teaching.

Faculty members from diverse backgrounds in education and experience, especially as related to their commitment to a specialty (e.g., pediatrics), strongly influence the outcome of the initial stage. In dealing with generalities, which are, in this case, rather abstract in nature, little real significance needs to be given to an individual faculty member's specific nursing interest. Generalizations must be the order of the day, for they constantly require the participants to relate their beliefs and thinking to those of a group. Each person's clinical expertise gives few overt rewards during this time. The identification of and commitment to realistic beliefs or truths within the philosophy, as well as the development of a theoretical framework, reflect the progress of the total faculty.

Most nursing educators have been unfamiliar with the development of the components involved in the directive stage, even though over the past two decades these same educators have succeeded in developing objectives and identifying teaching content. Lack of familiarity with such a framework and a sparsity of guidelines offer little upon which to build a sense of security for most faculty. This insecurity tends to create a "holding pattern" at the first stage of the curriculum process. It is not uncommon to find a faculty spending years developing a philosophy and a theoretical framework.

If the directive stage dictates curriculum decisions, it is reasonable to support the notion that once a faculty completes the first stage, most of the remaining stages can be developed by small groups or even, theoretically, by an individual. Although this may be true in a literal sense, all faculty members must be involved at every step in order to ensure commitment and implementation. If there is a well-stated philosophy, the remainder of the program will follow logically.

Formative Stage

The formative stage of the process has three components:

1. curriculum design and requirements
2. level and course objectives
3. content map

The formative stage requires the ability to develop more specificity and it gives meaning and form to the directive stage of the curriculum process. Now the curriculum design takes shape which leads to the development of level objectives for each year of the program. This, in turn, points to the creation of course descriptions and course objectives. Level and course objectives are later used in formative evaluations of the program. The content map is designed to show how the nursing courses will meet level and course objectives.

In this stage faculty members make decisions on the courses and learning experiences necessary to fulfill and carry out the imperatives of the directive stage. The total curriculum design is completed and provides a balance between and among university or college requirements for the degree, support courses for the major, nursing courses, and electives.

University or college requirements for a degree are generally specific and clearly defined. Support courses in the natural and social sciences and humanities are specified to reflect the nature of the philosophy and theoretical framework of the nursing program. Provisions for electives are also based on commitments made during the directive stage. Nursing courses are planned based on decisions made during the directive stage and the availability and use of support courses. Prerequisites to courses are identified and a logical design emerges.

The success or failure of the faculty in the development of the components in the formative stage is directly related to the faculty's achievements within the first stage. A carefully developed philosophy with a glossary of terms, theoretical framework, and characteristics of the graduate will ensure success in the development of the components in the formative stage. When difficulties are encountered, they are most likely due to the need to clarify some aspect of the curriculum components within the first stage. This point cannot be emphasized enough because it is when the faculty moves from one stage to the other that most problems are recognized.

In the development of objectives, a greater variety of literature sources and number of approaches is available to the faculty. There are definitive guidelines that can be used to restore a sense of security, of which many may have felt deprived during the initial stage. All too frequently faculty members have viewed the development of isolated objectives as the essence of the curriculum process leaving them with no direction as to how to utilize these objectives when the process is completed. It is only through the direction given the development of objectives during the directive stage that their usefulness and place within the educational system become identified. Too often these tend to be duplicative and nonprogressive (from course to course) as well as inadequate in their ability to differentiate learning.

Functional Stage

The functional stage consists of three components:

1. approaches to content
2. teaching methodology and learning experiences
3. validation of learning

This stage represents to most faculty members the action part of the curriculum process and it is generally considered the most relevant stage of the process. Now it is time to put into practice the components of the two previous stages. Sometimes this creates anxiety in faculty members who may find they have difficulty acting on their earlier decisions. Problems arise in the functional stage because flaws are discovered in prior decision making. Of course, such a discovery would demand a reexamination of previous findings. Therefore, it is essential to circulate adequate information while proceeding to reinforce the commitments made and to make clear at all times the prime purpose of the activities.

Until the whole curriculum begins to function, the course outlines may appear vague and often ill-defined. As each course is taught for the first time, the faculty and students will challenge approaches to content and compare their relationship to the developed curriculum. During this stage, total faculty cooperation will be necessary in order to ensure the appropriate development of the nursing courses that will follow.

The functional stage offers the faculty the opportunity to use the results of the directive and formative stages in a creative, personalized way. Whether the courses are individually or team taught, it is the responsibility of all faculty members to use their professional judgment in confirming what is truly viable. Their commitment is to assist students in meeting course objectives as identified in the formative stage, but their approaches can differ in terms of their priorities and instructional strengths. Tools are developed to validate learning and identify grades and used for evaluation of students. It is at this stage of the process where the greatest number of revisions can be made without disrupting the curriculum. Since the course objectives and course descriptions are the result of the decisions made during the formative stage and since at this stage improvements can be made without too much difficulty, altering approaches to teaching or testing as the courses evolve should facilitate the ease with which learning occurs. But there is a tendency when making decisions at this point to either revise the course objectives or not utilize them. Such a tendency becomes a serious problem for it can cause the deterioration of the entire curriculum by creating dysfunctional and disconnected learning experiences. This deterioration is more likely to occur when the faculty has not been involved in all stages of the process or when the faculty is unprepared educationally to use the curriculum process.

Once the approaches to content are developed, the other components of the functional stage can be developed simultaneously to ensure their interrelationship. During this development it is important that the faculty never loses sight of the decisions made during the directive stage. Constant reinforcements of the beliefs of faculty members as expressed in the philosophy will serve to strengthen their commitment and understanding. It is an opportune time to enhance clarity; minor revisions, therefore, can be made which illuminate the original intent. Obviously, any change that is seen as changing the original essence of the philosophy will require a complete analysis of how it affects the subsequent components. If faculty members work together during each stage and give serious thought to each component, substantive changes in philosophy will be rare or minimal.

Evaluative Stage

The evaluative stage, the last step in the curriculum process, consists of three components:

1. input

2. throughput

3. output

This stage represents an analysis of the degree of success of the curriculum design as it relates to the stated characteristics of the graduate who has completed the nursing program. It is the least understood stage of the curriculum process and it is frequently ignored. It must be clearly understood that what we are addressing here is an evaluation of the curriculum. The

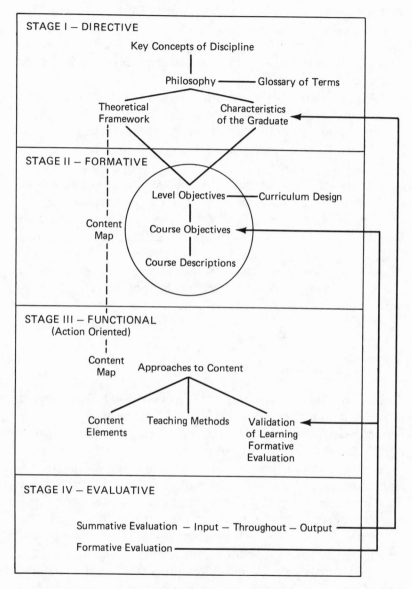

Figure   1.1
Conceptualization of the Curriculum Process

measure of success of the curriculum is the extent to which the graduates of the program meet the *characteristics of the graduate* operational at the time of their graduation. Diagnostic tools that measure the characteristics must be located or developed.

Input refers to the assessment of student characteristics at an early stage in their professional education. Throughput includes those activities that affect the students such as teaching, learning experiences, and grading. Output refers to the ability of the graduate to perform in relation to the desired characteristics. This supports the concept of learning which, fundamentally, means change. Students who enter the program do have a certain amount of knowledge, skills, and attitudes (input) that are affected by the educational process during the course of the program (throughput) and should be notably changed as they leave the program (output). Involved is the essence of change reflected in the concept of learning; throughput is measured against input and output characteristics.

Summary

The use of the curriculum process in curriculum development provides the faculty with a useful tool. The curriculum process is systematic, logical, dynamic, and spiraled in nature since it reflects all characteristics of a process. There are four stages in the curriculum process (directive, formative, functional, and evaluative) all of which blend together to form the image of a whole (see Fig. 1.1). Each stage gives guidance and direction to another stage and, in a sense, affirms the meaning of the other. There must be agreement and support between and among the stages so that the identification of the ideas within each of the parts of the curriculum process is consistent. If any one of the stages is not developed appropriately, the subsequent stages of the process will be weak and will provide little guidance. The total faculty must be involved in curriculum development to ensure commitment and implementation.

2

Directive Stage

The directive stage of the curriculum process, the first step in the process, is probably the most important stage since it lays the groundwork for all subsequent stages. It gives direction to the rest of the process. In this chapter the four components of this stage—the philosophy, the glossary of terms, the characteristics of the graduate, and the theoretical framework—are discussed, showing their relationships and consistency with one another.

The Philosophy

Philosophy is a way of viewing the whole of the world around us so that we can gain insights into reality. It is reflective of our knowledge about things in some comprehensive and logical way. Both the deductive and inductive processes of thinking are used to explain the nature of the whole. Values, ethics, and esthetics are crucial elements of philosophical thinking.

A philosophy for a nursing program is a way of viewing the world of nursing and nursing education: the nature of the discipline and the nature of teaching and learning.

For curriculum purposes, the characteristics of a philosophy mirror the study of philosophy in general. Therefore, philosophy

1. reflects abstract reasoning in relation to the whole;

2. considers the general nature of morals and makes choices about values and ideals;

3. identifies relationships between concepts and theories; and

4. uses logical rather than empirical approaches.

Thus, by definition, a curriculum philosophy is a speculative and analytical examination of beliefs which are logically conceptualized relating to a state of affairs. A curriculum philosophy integrates concepts, theories, and propositions about the "real world." For purposes of this discussion, some terms need to be defined.

Beliefs are accepted opinions or convictions of the truth that are not necessarily supported by scientific knowledge. Beliefs are useful in trying to discover what is common knowledge or what is commonly thought about a particular idea. Sometimes beliefs are found to be myths once they have been researched. However, beliefs are still useful in identifying areas of agreement among a group.

A *concept* has been referred to as an idea, an abstract notion. Chinn and Jacobs say that a concept is a "complex mental formulation of events, objects or properties which are derived from an individual's perceptual experience."[1] A concept provides a mental image about a phenomenon that can be further discussed, modified, and refined. For example, the

---

[1] P. L. Chinn, and M. K. Jacobs, "A Model for Theory Development in Nursing," *Advances in Nursing Science*, Vol. I, No. 1 (October, 1978), p. 5.

concept of a chair provides a mental image to most of us as something to sit on. But is it an armchair, a straight chair, a rocking chair, or a lounge chair? All are modifiers of the original concept, and for purposes of a group discussion one type of chair might be identified as key for purposes of limiting and focusing the discussion.

A *proposition* is a testable statement that shows a relationship between two or more concepts. Sometimes theories are defined in the same way; however a *theory* is a much more complex set of interrelationships between and among concepts, propositions, facts, principles and laws useful to predict, understand, and/or control phenomena.

Including a set of propositions in the philosophy enables faculty members to identify the theories and concepts that they must consider as giving direction and support to the selection of content and learning experiences.

For curriculum purposes, a statement of the program's philosophy gives the curriculum direction because it reflects the nature of the discipline of nursing and nursing education. Within the realm of the totality of nursing a philosophy integrates and synthesizes fundamental beliefs that are expressed about the discipline. A curriculum philosophy differs from a general statement of purposes or goals for a university in that the purpose of the curriculum philosophy is to *guide* the educational process of the learner in a particular field.

Purposes and Goals

The development of the philosophy needs to be seen in terms of its purpose and goal. The purpose, simply stated, is to direct the entire curriculum process with the goal of affecting every learning experience in which there is an interaction between the students and the world of knowledge. Such interactions facilitate learning and take innumerable forms within the educational environment. For example, classroom teaching, clinical laboratory experience, counseling and advising of students, evaluation forms, all speak to the educational process.

A philosophical statement that is easily misunderstood, ambiguously written, or viewed as nondirective is truly a total waste of time and effort. If on one end of the vertical continuum of the curriculum process we place the philosophy and on the other end we place the learning experiences, either the deductive or the inductive reasoning approach should lead us to the same conclusions. For example, if the faculty believes that human beings have dignity, then the learning experiences should be built on this belief. Reviewing either the philosophy deductively or the learning experiences inductively should lead to similar conclusions.

Nursing education occurs within specific environments. Therefore, faculty members must keep in mind the goals of their institution when they build their philosophical statements. For example, within a university a frequently stated goal is to provide an environment conducive to the search for new knowledge through research activities. As a result, nursing must reflect a commitment to the notion of the advancement of knowledge. A nursing program's philosophical statements need not reiterate the goals of the parent institution, but they should be utilized as a guide in developing the program.

In developing a philosophy a faculty should take the following steps:

1. identify key concepts;

2. discuss specific beliefs about each concept;

3. show relationships between and among the concepts and an ordering among concepts;

4. develop propositions.

Identification of Key Concepts

The faculty must conceptualize about the discipline of nursing and nursing education. This means that faculty members must have time to sit and discuss with each other their beliefs (views, ideas, opinions) about nursing. Beliefs are regarded here as accepted opinions or convictions of the truth that are not based on positive knowledge. These beliefs should be recorded and reviewed by the faculty until the major or key concepts can be identified and agreed upon. It is not possible or appropriate to deal with the totality of beliefs. Emphasis is given to those that give meaning to the discipline, make sense to all members of the faculty, fit with the university or institutional goals, and give direction to subsequent decision making in the curriculum process. The faculty uses deductive thinking to arrive at the four or five key concepts with which they will deal.

A nursing program faculty in a university founded on a specific religious orientation would have difficulty in promoting a philosophy that was in direct conflict with the university's stated ideology. Conversely, a nursing program in a state university would have difficulty promulgating a philosophy espousing beliefs specific to a particular religious viewpoint. The faculties of both institutions, whatever their personal beliefs, would identify key concepts that are acceptable to all.

What a faculty strives for is a consensus that a particular belief is necessary to the practice of nursing. The faculty must recognize the fact that while some beliefs may be important in a personal or religious context, they may not be essential in a nursing context.

Some common beliefs about the notion of nursing include the following:

Nursing is a practice discipline.

It involves a service to human beings.

Human beings exist within a society.

Nursing provides care and nurturance to human beings.

Human beings are entitled to respect and dignity.

A society has common interests and goals.

The discipline focuses on health.

Nursing involves health promotion and maintenance.

Health is the right of everyone in society.

Nursing is humanitarian.

Society should be responsive to the needs of human beings.

A quick review of these statements indicates that nursing, human beings, society, and health can be identified as key concepts. They are referred to more than once in different ways and they show a faculty's concern for the concepts.

In a real-world situation, faculty members would elaborate on and list their beliefs, no matter how redundant, until a pattern begins to emerge. Then the key concepts would be extrapolated from the listed beliefs. If an idea or notion were referred to over and over again in many different ways, it would be worthy of consideration. Something that is mentioned only once or twice may be discarded.

Thus, in the development of a philosophy, the faculty must identify the basic beliefs, values, and ideas essential to the practice of nursing. From these will evolve the logical concepts that give meaning to the discipline.

Beliefs about Each Concept

The second step the faculty takes in developing a philosophy is to discuss their specific beliefs about each concept. This is different from what was done initially in stating broad and general beliefs about nursing and identifying the key concepts from recurring themes in the belief. Now the faculty is further refining and specifying beliefs about a concept; it is getting down to the core ideas. For example, human beings was identified as a key concept because of the beliefs initially stated about nursing in general. Now the faculty is looking precisely at its specific beliefs about human beings. These beliefs are recorded, reviewed, and refined. Some of them are discarded. A consensus on the beliefs is reached and agreed upon by the faculty. At the same time a logical sense of ordering takes place. This is not to be construed as setting priorities.

Number one is not considered most important; it is considered most logical in the sequencing of ideas about each concept.

Relationships and Ordering
among the Concepts

The third step the faculty takes in developing a philosophy is to show relationships between and among the concepts and an ordering among concepts. The relation or interactive nature between and among concepts may vary depending on the ordering of the concepts. It is useful for a faculty to conceptualize a model that reflects how the concepts relate to each other. This pictorial image may take a variety of forms depending on the ordering given to the concepts by the group. Figure 2.1a shows human beings as related to health within the environment and nursing as the unifying concepts. Another possibility would be to view human beings as the core concept around which the other three concepts are developed (see Fig. 2.1b). Many alternative visual approaches are possible and logical to the discipline. Such conceptualizations give clues to the further development of a philosophical statement since they give order to the thinking process.

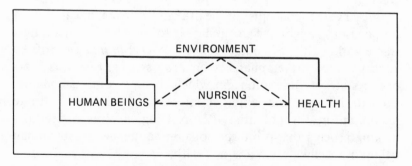

Figure 2.1a
Model of Human Beings as Related to Health
within the Environment

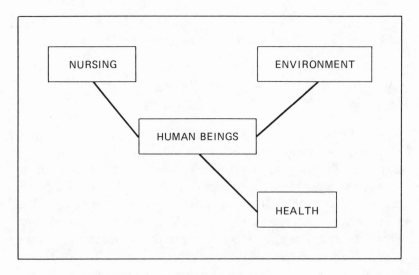

Figure 2.1b
Model of Human Beings as the Core Concept

Developing Propositions

After identifying the key *concepts* related to the discipline and establishing some ordering in terms of logical sequencing, then it is useful for the faculty to take the fourth step: develop propositions that reflect a state of affairs about a specific concept.

Using the concepts of health and nursing the following propositions might be formulated to develop a theoretical framework. (This, of course, reflects a *very limited view* of the concept since the emphasis is on process.) (1) Health is a dynamic state of functioning in which there is continual adaptation to internal and external stresses in order to facilitate maximum health potential. (2) Nursing involves a decision-making process that is interpersonal in nature and assists human beings in reaching their goal of health.

As the faculty continues to expand on its beliefs in relation to each of the concepts, the philosophical statement begins to take form. Efforts need to be made so that the propositions integrate one concept with another and build on the previous propositions. During this activity, it is essential that all propositions be reviewed on the grounds of their validity from a philosophical position. Measures of validity include intuition and observations that reflect professional experiences, analysis and conceptualization of knowledge giving logical inferences to beliefs, and the acceptance of authority for greater objectivity.[2] Validity must be questioned when emotions, traditions, or rationalizations influence decisions. "Bandwagoning ideas" must be carefully assessed for validity in terms of whether they emerged from inference and analysis or from false ideological thinking. Although this is not an easy task, utilizing the principles of reasoning will ensure a greater degree of validity. This includes emphasizing the relationships and the consistency between each proposition.

After the philosophy has been developed to reflect the key concepts of the discipline of nursing, the faculty must develop propositions about the concept of learning. It is through the development and identification of the faculty's beliefs about learning that recognition will be given to the approach to teaching that needs to emerge. Beliefs about the learner lead to assumptions based on the theories of learning which in turn generate propositions that will affect the process of education.

The ability of the faculty to develop a curriculum philosophy is strongly influenced by its ability to deal with abstractions and to conceptualize its beliefs in some orderly fashion. The greater the faculty's theoretical base of knowledge, the stronger the philosophical statement will be. Leaders will emerge from those who have a greater knowledge of the concepts. The knowledge base of the faculty needs to be carefully assessed and, for most groups, additional learning will need to take place prior to or parallel with curriculum development activities.

Even if there is a strong theoretical base, faculty members need to be able to reach a consensus on their beliefs in terms

---

[2] Henry Leonard, *Principles of Reasoning and Introduction To: Logic Methodology and the Theory of Signs* (New York: Dover Publications, 1967), p. 71.

Confidence	Doubt	Confidence
−10	0	+10
Complete Rejection	Indecision	Complete Acceptance

Figure 2.2
Belief Scale

of their validity. Communication and interactive skills are important so that doubts versus acceptance of each other's ideas will evolve. As belief statements emerge from each concept, general acceptance or rejection needs to be discussed on the basis of a continuum similarly approached by Leonard.[3] By using a belief scale of + or − 10 with 0 representing real or total indecision or doubt, it is possible to identify the most rational significant beliefs/attitudes of the group (see Fig. 2.2). The closer to the positive confidence point on the scale, the more likely that beliefs will emerge that will be truly functional for the further development of the curriculum. Negative confidence rules out the inclusion of certain belief statements. These, by their omission, become significant to the educational process. The faculty must be cognizant that the philosophy dictates the educational process and, thus, a commitment to it is essential.

A philosophy for a nursing program, then, is based upon the institution's stated philosophy, purposes, or goals. The philosophy includes propositions about the four or five key concepts a faculty has identified as the characteristics of the nature of nursing. It lays the groundwork for the subsequent development of the curriculum.

---

[3] Henry Leonard, *Principles of Reasoning* (New York: Dover Publications, 1967), pp. 49–55.

Glossary of Terms

A glossary is a list of terms which are defined specific to a special field. A glossary of terms is always helpful in a document that is to be used as a guiding or foundational force. The faculty must define how terms are being used in the context of the faculty's philosophy. Sometimes even words that appear to be universal in meaning need to be defined for clarity or specificity.

Deductive in nature, abstract thinking becomes increasingly more specific. As the process evolves, greater clarity should follow, especially in the use of language. Discussion tends to center around the meaning of specific words. Such words need to be identified as the philosophy is developed and they need to be given particular meaning by the faculty. A glossary of terms is essential so that a common frame of reference can be developed by the group which will facilitate more effective communication. The term *society* would seem to have a universal meaning, but it needs to be defined relative to its use in a particular program's philosophy. It can be defined or limited by geographic parameters, common goals or views, special interests, and so forth. The same goes for the term *health*. Does it mean the absence of illness or does it mean a dynamic state of well-being?

The purpose of the glossary of terms is to make very clear how the faculty defines the particular terms it is using. This in and of itself helps to give guidance to students and faculty since it clearly indicates what is meant when speaking to the terms in the philosophy.

Theoretical Framework

A theoretical framework is developed from a curriculum philosophy for the purpose of identifying and structuring the content of the educational process. *Theoretical* in this context is used to identify the content elements and framework and to reorganize the structure of those elements. The *content elements* include concepts, theories, knowledge, propositions, skills, and attitudes. In relation to the discipline of nursing, the framework includes the *content* and *process* essential for the practice of nursing. Content is reflective of the theoretical knowledge base and process is the use of that knowledge for practice. For example, the knowledge gained through an understanding of health is utilized within the context of the nursing process. Thus, a theoretical framework is a structure made up of content elements identified from the philosophy and united in such a way as to give sequence to the learning activities. The integration of such content gives the curriculum a sense of the whole so that a complete view of the knowledge, skills, and attitudes to be achieved by the learner can be identified. Without this essential component of the curriculum process, there is little or no chance that the philosophy will be implemented into each learning and evaluative experience. It is during the directive stage that the faculty member makes most of the significant decisions on the "what" and "how" of the practice of nursing will be taught.

Content Elements

In order to facilitate the orderly development of the theoretical framework, the framework must be viewed as a deductive process based on the curriculum philosophy with all of its stated propositions.

Thus, each proposition within the philosophy is used to identify the *content elements* and a structure is developed which provides for the sequence of learning that reflects those content elements. With a greater degree of specificity, the content elements will evolve so that relationships can be found among and within the key concepts. This will later lead to the grouping of certain content elements so that an integrative approach to teaching can occur.

Content elements should not be viewed as identical in

meaning. Knowledge usually means facts and includes scientific principles which have been empirically studied. Theories assist in the creation of new knowledge but may not have been adequately researched. The difference between knowledge and theory is not always clear since within various disciplines the definitions of these terms differ. Theories may often be included as components of knowledge, but all theories do not reflect knowledge. Skills involve practice as performance activities and are generally built on a knowledge or theoretical base. Attitudes reflect a position in relation to a person or thing. Thus, in deducting from propositions all of these content elements must be identified.

Sequencing of Content

Content elements should be seen in the context of the entire curriculum offerings and not just in relation to the nursing requirements. Thus, it is necessary for the faculty to identify early what elements will be included in the supporting, general education, or nursing courses. Such decisions will be made during the formative stage of the curriculum process within the curriculum design. For example, if a proposition speaks to developmental theory as a content element, the faculty can decide to (1) require a course in developmental psychology and build on the content, (2) place such content within the nursing courses, or (3) require a course in developmental psychology and expand on the theoretical base offered within the nursing courses. The third point is usually most feasible since prerequisite courses such as this one usually do not offer developmental theories for the entire life span and tend to view human beings in a narrow way.

The sequencing of content should reflect the logic of inquiry in relation to the learner. Implied in sequencing is the use of prerequisite content at each step of the educational process. When content is viewed as isolated pieces of information that require little or no previous knowledge, it can be taught in a nonprogressive oriented curriculum structure. Such an approach usually cannot deal with an integrative and generalized approach to teaching since it emphasizes isolated facts that are not ordered to show such relationships. This is usually true of the "medical model" curriculum in which students are taught diseases with little or no relationship between the states of pathology or the totality of the client. The sequencing to this approach is usually limited to the sciences as prerequisite to nursing content. But within the nursing offerings there is little or no demand for prerequisite content reflecting a nonlogical approach to the learning activities.

Sequencing of content should also reflect the level of difficulty that is required in the use of that content for practice. Content which is more easily internalized, or in which the individual's past experience would assist in learning, or which is projected to be most frequently utilized within the discipline and requires a lot of practice should be identified and taught early. Similarly, content that requires a greater degree of synthesis involving a breadth of knowledge should be offered near the end. Here the developmental level of the student must be considered based on the philosophical proposition about learning.

The arranging or ordering of content elements requires some recognition that theories and knowledge can have a different order of generality. For example, would communication, interactive, and interpersonal theories be viewed as having the same level of generality or should interpersonal theory reflect a broad theoretical approach in which interactive or communication theory would be viewed more narrowly? The relationship and breadth of each theory needs to be assessed to determine the approach to content. The question of generality or specificity is a difficult one unless the propositions within the philosophy are used as guidelines. If nursing is viewed as an interpersonal process, the conclusion could be drawn that indeed communication and interactive theories need to be viewed as having greater specificity than interpersonal theories. Again, this is a reflection of the dictates of the philosophy.

Horizontal and Vertical Strands

Within the context of progressive learning and the sequence of content elements, it is helpful to identify the strands or threads that can be utilized to order that content. Strands can be viewed as *vertical* or *horizontal.* *Vertical* strands are used to identify *content* areas such as concepts, theories, and knowledge that are broadly conceived and give meaning to the building of content. *Horizontal* strands are constant and *process* oriented and focus on the use of the content. It is the interaction between vertical strands—the content—and the horizontal strands—the process—that explains the discipline (see Fig. 2.3).

Leadership theory can be viewed as a vertical strand and decision making, a component of leadership, can be viewed as a horizontal strand.

Since vertical strands are progressive and build on previous content areas, they are the key to the identification of different levels within the educational process.

These strands require that the content elements be viewed broadly in terms of a *continuum.* This approach provides direction for the placement of learning experiences. A continuum connects content that can be moved forward and reflects a sequence. For example, in Fig. 2.3 leadership could have been viewed as a continuum with content elements related to coordination and change as shown in Fig. 2.4. This continuum approach requires that the learning experience be *initially* focused on the content elements related to coordination within a decision-making framework followed by those related to change in decision making.

Educational programs which are two, three, or four years in length must identify the content elements that will be emphasized at different time periods. Thus, in setting up the theoretical framework, the entire length of the program must be identified. Generally, it is only during the clinical portion of the program that the horizontal strands are identified. This is acceptable since process reflects the practice of the discipline which is built on a knowledge base. It needs to be recognized

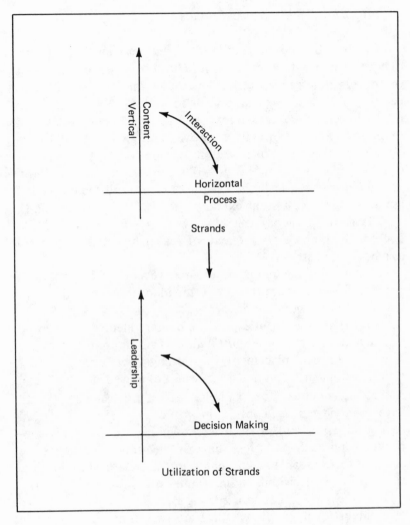

Figure 2.3
Relationship of Vertical and Horizontal Strands

that these strands which reflect a process are also based on other content elements. For example, decision making and interactive theories are essential to the use of the nursing process. Thus, the faculty must decide whether or not to offer

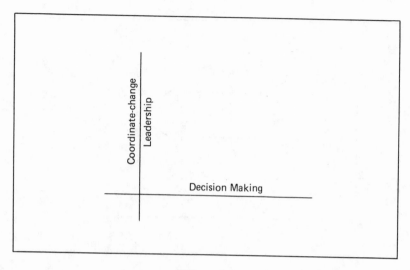

Figure 2.4

Vertical Strands on a Continuum

such content elements within a foundation course in nursing prerequisite to process strands. For example, within a four-year program that offers clinical courses in the third and fourth years, the process-oriented strands—horizontal in nature—would be identified during the second half of the program. Since the content elements such as theories and knowledge are given throughout the curriculum, they must be identified for the entire four years. The structure of the framework could be developed as shown in Fig. 2.5.

Since the horizontal strands are a constant, they would be the same for both the third and fourth years of the program. It is especially important that the vertical strands for the third and fourth years which reflect the major portion of the nursing content be clearly developed. As a matter of fact, almost all of the content offered within the first two years is offered by the faculty teaching the supportive courses which are discipline oriented and not too integrated. It becomes a main function of the theoretical framework to integrate and utilize such content later (see Fig. 2.6).

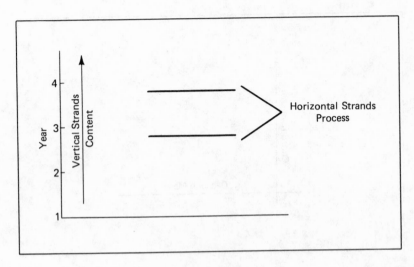

Figure 2.5
Structure of the Framework

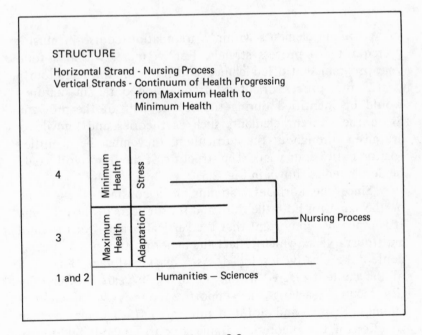

Figure 2.6
Levels within the Framework

Characteristics of the Graduate

The characteristics of the graduate reflect those behaviors which are expected of the graduate at the end of the program of study. They are not terminal in nature but a foundation for practice that will be used to further develop the practitioner. The characteristics reflect the theoretical framework in that they contain the content and process essential for practice but are expressed in terms of behavioral objectives. These will later be used to develop level and course objectives during the formative stage of the curriculum process. Thus, the characteristics of the graduate can be defined as those broad behaviors that mirror the philosophy in its content and process and that contain the highest level of achievement of the new graduate. Within this definition are some important components:

1. Broad behaviors are developed from the propositions in relation to all the concepts that relate to the discipline. Unless this is done, there is no way of ensuring that the philosophy will be implemented. The development of characteristics which are not clearly inherent within the philosophy will misdirect the learning experiences. Similarly, if clearly stated propositions do not lead to objectives, then large vacuums will appear within the curriculum.

2. Since the characteristics of the graduate will later be used in conjunction with the theoretical framework to develop more specific objectives, essential theoretical knowledge, skills, and attitudes need to be identified. Also, since learning is progressive and builds on one level after the other, the highest level of achievement is identified with each characteristic. Such levels may be identified by using a taxonomy such as Bloom's or by the faculty in conjunction with its beliefs about learning.

The National League for Nursing and the American Nurses Association have developed or are developing characteristics for all types of nursing programs. These may be useful for discussion but it needs to be recognized that since they were developed without a statement of philosophy, it would not be appropriate for a particular program to utilize them as their program characteristics. However, it is helpful to compare and contrast them with those developed within a program since they do reflect common beliefs about the graduates of the differing types of nursing programs.

The following characteristic of the baccalaureate graduate will be used to demonstrate each component of the definition.

Utilize the leadership skills through involvement
with others in meeting health needs and nursing goals.[4]

Philosophical Bases

Inherent in the characteristic are certain philosophical statements. For example:
Human beings have health needs which relate to nursing goals.
Nursing leadership involves functioning with others.
Health needs can be met through the use of leadership skills.

Content and Process

Specific content that can be identified relate to knowledge about leadership, health, needs, and nursing. Process includes skills in leadership and the identification of nursing goals such as those developed within the context of the nursing process.

Level of Achievement

The highest level of achievement identified is in the process area related to the application of leadership skill.

---

[4] *Characteristics of Baccalaureate Education Nursing.* Division of baccalaureate and higher degree programs, New York National League for Nursing, 1979 p. 3, Pub No. 15-1758.

The characteristics, as a total package, are the summation of all of the behaviors of the graduate. While they need to be quite broad in their language, difficulties will arise if they are overdeveloped and contain too much content and process. For example, the following characteristic (uses leadership skills and nursing theories within the context of the nursing process to meet the health needs of individuals and groups, and identify gaps in community health programs) is overdeveloped. Therefore it would be better to divide it into two separate parts, as described below.

CHARACTERISTIC	CONTENT AND PROCESS COMPONENTS
1. Utilizes *nursing theories* within the context of the *nursing process* to meet *health needs* of *individuals* and *groups.*	Nursing theories Nursing process Health needs Individuals and groups
2. Uses *leadership* skills to *enable others* to identify gaps in *community health programs.*	Leadership theory Leadership skills Health systems Community needs Interpersonal skills

The theoretical framework and the characteristics of the graduate are reflective of the philosophy. They are developed to support one another during the other stages of the curriculum process. Although they both identify the content and the process of the philosophy, the theoretical framework focuses on structure for sequencing learning while the characteristics of the graduate identify a level of behavior. This relationship is helpful in providing the idea of a "check and balance" system during the directive stage. Both content and process components can be checked for consistency within and between the philosophy, theoretical framework, and characteristics. The terminology used must be defined in the glossary unless the meanings of the words are universally clear and acceptable.

Summary

The directive stage of the curriculum process consists of four components: the philosophy, the glossary of terms, the characteristics of the graduate, and the theoretical framework. In the directive stage the faculty lays the foundation for all subsequent activities related to curriculum development. It is in this stage that decisions are made about the discipline of nursing and the teaching/learning process which give direction to all other decisions relative to curriculum. By consensus, the faculty will control and manage in a rather authoritative way the later stages of the curriculum process.

3

Formative Stage

The formative stage essentially is the "bridge between the directive and functional stages" of the curriculum process. The generalizations developed during the directive stage will be drawn in such a way as to impact on the components of the functional stage such as learning experiences.

During this stage, constant reference must be made to all of the components of the directive stage. At this point, minor revisions are often made of statements in the philosophy to increase clarity. Such changes usually clarify the previous thinking of the faculty rather than modify previously developed propositions. Such a process of reasoning needs to be viewed as continuous since a curriculum evolves and is dynamic rather than static. Careful consideration and recognition are essential as to whether changes reflect clarification or modification. Modification requires a complete assessment of its impact on all the components of the curriculum process while clarification enhances the understanding of previously developed statements.

The formative stage of the curriculum process consists of three components:

1. curriculum design and requirements
2. level and course objectives
3. content map

The curriculum design identifies and sequences course requirements so that learning experiences are structured throughout the program. The level and course objectives mirror the characteristics and give meaning to the strands within the theoretical framework. They reflect the changes in behavior expected of the student at a given point in time within the program, usually at the end of a year. Course objectives reflect the level objectives and are more specific and detailed in construction. The relationship between each of these components is one of deduction and further clarification. For example, the course objectives further explain the meaning of the level objective and theoretical framework. The content map gives direction to course planning and teaching.

Curriculum Design

The plan and form of the curriculum design is primarily based on the structure of the total curriculum package. The total course requirements need to develop within a framework that is reflective of the specific institutional requirements for the degree and the philosophy of the program. Guidelines to follow include:

1. The total structure of the design should reflect the discipline. Nursing as a professional field is involved primarily in a practice or process model which is different from a liberal arts discipline which tends to be more content oriented.

2. The philosophical propositions, especially those related to nursing and learning, should be viewed as guidelines.

3. The curriculum package should include general education and the humanities, supporting courses, and nursing. These three areas should be fairly well balanced.

4. The designated sequence of all courses should take into account the level of knowledge necessary to enter a particular course. The vertical strands within the theoretical framework will have the greatest impact on such sequencing.

5. The resources available within the institution in terms of available course offerings should be assessed.

6. A clear distinction should be made between nursing and other knowledge in order to identify appropriate supporting courses. This is especially true in relation to science requirements.

A variety of designs such as seen in Fig. 3.1 are feasible in terms of course requirements. Ideally, such designs should facilitate and enhance learning experiences at each level and be as flexible as possible to allow for individual differences. Because of the limitations on clinical and physical resources, the planned organized use of faculty throughout the academic year, and the ordering of content in a very progressive way, there is often little flexibility in curriculum requirements. Thus, in the development of the design, the faculty should be cognizant of this built-in rigidity and identify ways to reduce it whenever possible. Flexibility is enhanced by allowing for many free electives and by limiting prerequisites to nursing courses unless found essential.

Curriculum models differ in their placement of the nursing major within the total requirements. In a building design, general education and supporting courses (such as the sciences) are generally required during the first two years of a four-year program (see Fig. 3.1a). In the last two years the nursing

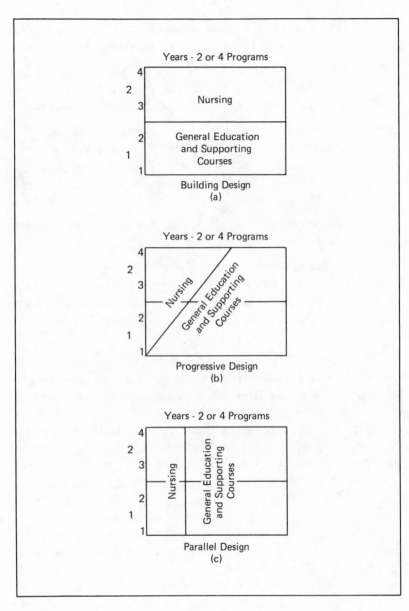

Figure 3.1
Models for Curriculum Designs

courses *build* on the previously acquired knowledge. Another approach, the progressive design, requires mostly general education and supporting courses early in the curriculum but add a limited number of nursing courses during the first two years (see Fig. 3.1b). This approach usually limits the content of the initial nursing courses to ones that do not require a strong base in the supporting courses. As the curriculum progressively develops, nursing requirements increase and others decrease. A design can also be developed that requires the same amount of nursing requirements throughout the four years (see Fig. 3.1c). Inherent in this model is a *parallel* approach to nursing and other requirements that build together to achieve an end. It should be noted that the building design and the progressive design are more cost effective for B.S.N. programs since faculty are primarily teaching in the last two years of the program. Having faculty, especially in clinical courses, spread out over three or four years increases the cost because more faculty members are generally needed.

The appropriate model selected for a particular nursing program should reflect the philosophy of the program. For example, inherent within the philosophy are propositions that speak to the basis of nursing practice and learning. The building design speaks strongly to nursing knowledge built on a strong educational, especially scientific, base. The progressive design focuses on much of the same commitment but not so rigidly. In contrast, the parallel design supports the idea that both nursing and other knowledges should be integrated throughout the program. What is significant in the selection of a model, or combination of them, is that the faculty has a rationale for the design. This is important so that the sequencing of course requirements can be *truly* reflective of the philosophy.

The philosophical propositions dictate what supporting and general education courses will be required. In reviewing the following statements, it becomes clear as to which among potentially hundreds of courses will be required of the nursing major.

PHILOSOPHICAL PROPOSITION	POTENTIAL COURSE REQUIREMENTS
Social change involves the interaction of political and social forces which affect an individual's cultural values.	Sociology Political Science Anthropology
Health is influenced by human beings' inherent capabilities as well as their potential for growth and development.	Biology; Genetics Psychology; Growth and development

The faculty must recognize that there is a limit to the number of courses that can be required for the degree. This limit should be reflective of the degree limits placed on other programs within the educational institution. Thus priorities must be established and vacuums must be identified for possible inclusion within some of the nursing content. For example, if the faculty believes that knowledge of nutrition is essential for the nursing major and such courses are not offered and are not going to be offered within the institution, the nursing faculty must account for this knowledge within the nursing courses.

Within any educational program there has to be a balance among the requirements essential for the degree, and the requirements essential for the major, and the requirements that are supportive of the major. It is the combination and integration of these requirements that give breadth to the educational process. Generally, the nursing faculty has difficulty in recognizing the value of a balanced curriculum package and tends to require too few general education courses, such as those in the humanities, and too many nursing and science courses. It is in those areas of knowledge with which faculty members are most familiar that they tend to require the greatest amount of content. One needs to refer back to the philosophy and theoretical framework for guidance. An appropriate balance should provide for approximately one-third of the requirements to be in general education and humanities, one-third in supporting courses (including sciences), and one-third in nursing courses. Also, within these requirements there should be some flexibility between and among courses and there should be provision for a number of free electives. Course requirements in the areas of religion, political science, or anthropology should allow the student to select among many course offerings rather than a specific one in any area. This is usually possible when the nursing content requires a broad theoretical base within a particular area rather than within specific content. Specific science courses such as anatomy should give the student information on the anatomy of human beings in totality rather than focus on a particular system of the body. Thus, the flexibility within a discipline is usually decreased in specific science courses.

The sequencing of requirements, especially the supporting sciences, is generally established by the faculty teaching those courses. As a result, such information must be available to the members of the nursing faculty as they develop the curriculum design. For example, biology and chemistry may be prerequisites to anatomy and physiology, or general psychology may be required before developmental or abnormal psychology can be taken. Thus, parallel to developing the curriculum design, specific course requirements, including those in the nursing major, must have the prerequisites clearly identified. This is a particularly important point. If nursing faculty members do not take it into consideration, they will find themselves teaching the content of other disciplines for which they are not prepared.

In addition to finding the appropriate proportion of the three areas of study—general education, supporting, and nursing courses—to develop the curriculum package, the faculty must be cognizant of the balance essential during each study period, such as a quarter or semester. For example, requiring three science courses with laboratory experiences within a given period—semester—can make it very difficult for many students to achieve their highest level of learning for that period of time. Ideally, most semesters should require approximately one-eighth and most quarters should require one-twelfth of a total curriculum package in a two- or four-year program.

Level and Course Objectives

Essentially, the development of level and course objectives represents a logical deductive process for the purpose of making broadly conceived characteristics more functional. In order to ensure a sense of order to the process, the strands identified within the theoretical framework become directive.

Level objectives are derived from the characteristics of the graduate and are reflective of the theoretical framework. They make explicit an expected change in the learner at an identified point in time within the total program which allows for cumulative learning. Generally, level objectives are formulated for each year of the program. Faculty can then say at the end of the first year students will be expected to meet one set of level objectives, at the end of the second year they will be expected to meet a second set of level objectives, and so on for each year of the program.

Level objectives provide both faculty and students with cumulative goals to be achieved. Level objectives are also useful for curriculum evaluation. They show the sequencing in learning and building that should occur within a given period of time.

As in the development of the characteristics, level and course objectives contain (1) the level of achievement expected at any given point within the program, (2) the identification of content from the vertical strands, and (3) a process component from the horizontal strands. At this point in the development of the curriculum, any weakness within the characteristics, glossary of terms, or theoretical framework will become obvious and will require some reassessment of the components that were developed during the directive stage.

Nursing course objectives are derived from the level objectives. They set the parameters for learning for a specific time period, e.g., one course which usually takes place during one quarter or one semester. It is possible that the specific time period could be a module in a course limiting the time frame to less than the quarter or semester course. Occasionally, course work involves more than the usual quarter or semester. For whatever time period, the course objectives set the parameters.

The following characteristic is used to show the development of level and course objectives. Additional strands are incorporated into the course objectives.

Example:

Characteristic. Evaluate selected research studies for the applicability of findings in the nursing process (see Fig. 3.2).

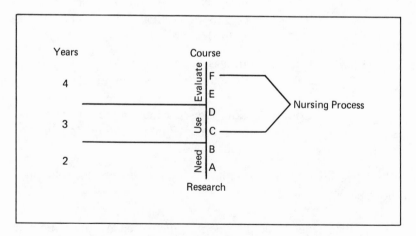

Figure 3.2
Vertical Strand—Research is on Three Levels:
Need, Use, and Evaluate. Horizontal Strand—
Nursing Process is on Two Levels.

Level objectives. Level objectives use the breakdown as identified on the vertical strand.

> Level
> 2—Understand the *need* for nursing research
> 3—*Use* research to provide nursing care
> 4—*Evaluate* research findings for use in providing nursing care

Course Objectives. Course objectives further delineate the focus of each course under each level if there is more than one nursing course.

> Level 2—Course a—Knows the various research methods
> Course b—Identifies the importance of nursing research in giving nursing care
>
> Level 3—Course c—Uses nursing research in the care of healthy individuals
> Course d—Uses nursing research in the care of individuals with long-term problems (the above objectives assume a vertical strand relating to health)
>
> Level 4—Course e—Judges research on the basis of its significance to individual client care
> Course f—Compares various research findings for use in providing nursing care

In reviewing the example, one should note the following about each course objective:

1. The level of achievement is identified by the expected behavior, such as knows, identifies, uses, judges, compares.

2. The content within each objective stems from the breakdown of the vertical strands.

3. The nursing process, a horizontal strand, is identified during the last two levels so that the first two courses (a and b) involve content instead of process.

The result of integrating the various strands and characteristics will lead to a package of course objectives that will influence all learning experiences.

Content Map

A useful way of dealing with content elements is to develop a content map. In a literal sense, a content map briefly outlines where you have been and where you are going. It also gives an indication of where you may end if you go off course. The development of a content map helps to facilitate the faculty's ability to identify the content elements in an appropriate sequence and it offers an opportunity to provide some balance throughout the nursing courses. This is a helpful step since all too frequently most of the content elements tend to be taught early in the program. The content map should include the major focus and the content elements of each of the clinical nursing courses as dictated by the components of the directive stage of the curriculum process.

The development of a content map is well worth the time and effort. It is an effective method of encouraging a large group of faculty members to be accountable for the content elements that are taught throughout the program. Thus, the content map accomplishes the following:

1. identifies the specific content elements that should be taught within each course;

2. allows the faculty to better understand what the students were previously taught, thus facilitating building the content in a progressive manner;

3. gives the faculty and students a sense of direction because it shows which content elements will follow;

4. gives structure to the differentiation of content elements from one course to another; and

5. assists in recognizing content areas not previously identified.

A sample content map is given in Table 3.1.

Course Outlines

A course outline leads the faculty and students to the approach to a particular course. In a sense, a course outline is a contractual agreement between teacher and student that facilitates the learner in meeting the stated objectives. In order to be useful, the course outline should be developed prior to the first class for discussion and review by students. It contains the course description, objectives of the course, content elements, and teaching and evaluative methods to be used and it also identifies their relationships. In other words, the course outline reflects a summation of the components within the formative and functional stages of the curriculum process. If specific directions and developed relationships are not outlined, neither the faculty nor the students will know what to expect.

A useful format for a course outline is as follows: Course description with dates, prerequisites, and the identification of faculty and their availability.

COURSE OBJECTIVES	CONTENT ELEMENTS IN SEQUENCE	TEACHING METHODS	EVALUATION METHODS
List all objectives in order of priority	Include areas identified with content map	Include classroom, independent and laboratory experiences	Identify tools used and due dates

Table 3.1
Sample Content Map (Content Elements)

FOCUS	NURSING I: Individual in a Maximum State of Health	NURSING II: Individual with Chronic Health Problems
Concepts and theories	Wellness Roger's theory Orlando's theory Etc.	Stress Roy's theory Vulnerability Etc.
Major content areas	Nursing process with healthy individuals Health promotion and protection Teaching Etc.	Nursing process with clients who are chronically ill Health care delivery system Poverty Etc.
Learning experiences	Health history Assessment skills Nursing process in unstructured settings Teaching as implementation strategy Etc.	Nursing process with clients in nursing homes and other long-term care settings Observations of multiple health care settings Etc.

The following reflect the rationale for the format and sequence of items identified within the course outline:

1. *Supports the curriculum process.* The course objectives evolved from the characteristics of the graduate

and level objectives. The content map was developed from the theoretical framework. Thus, in the same manner, the course objectives should assist in sequencing the content elements in order to identify the most appropriate teaching and evaluative methods.

2. *Identifies the relationship between the parts.* Since the objectives and content elements tend to change less frequently, it is the teaching and evaluation methods that change most often. Thus, their relationships must be clearly established; otherwise, with time, they will not be appropriate. This is especially true when there is inadequate time planned.

3. *Clarifies the similarities and differences between the components.* Frequently there is confusion about the similarities and differences between teaching and evaluation methods. For example, required or recommended readings or experiences are teaching methods in terms of their major purpose, but, admittedly, they can be used later to develop written test items. Term papers are both a teaching method reflective of an independent activity to facilitate certain behaviors and an evaluative method in that they are graded. It is important that the rationale for the selection of teaching methods support the development of specific criteria for grading. It is essential that the learner understand the difference between a learning activity and an evaluative activity, especially in the clinical area.

4. *Provides for emphasis through prioritization.* Although all course objectives must be met by the learner at some minimum level of achievement, the faculty needs to prioritize them as a way of giving greater emphasis on or focus within the course. Prioritization requires sound professional judgment on the part of the faculty. This approach offers the learner the ability to spend a

greater degree of time and effort in those areas that are of greater consequence than others.

5. *Identifies sequence of content elements.* Since the course objectives are placed in order of emphasis, the content elements will be identified in that context. It is essential that these elements also reflect progressive learning and be sequenced in terms of the foundational or basic elements being offered first. This may require some readjustments of integration. Also, certain content elements may easily relate to more than one objective. This needs to be recognized and viewed as a building process. Thus, only the additional content should be offered at a later time.

6. *Offers a view of the totality for curriculum assessment.* Combining all aspects of a course provides the faculty and the learner with a sense of the "whole." This allows them to view each course as a package and evaluate it in terms of its thoroughness, clarity of purpose, and relationship with the entire curriculum. When course outlines are similarly developed throughout the program, they should assist the faculty in inductively reevaluating their developed curriculum. Thus, in combination, all course outlines can be viewed in terms of their relationships to the theoretical framework, characteristics of the graduate, and the philosophy. The course outline provides a check and balance system to keep the curriculum more viable.

It is helpful if individual faculty members attempt to develop the course outline individually prior to the group meeting. This will not only facilitate group interactions but also the process.

The development of an appropriate course outline is not an easy task and should be done in a sequence supportive of the curriculum process. Thus, the following steps are useful:

STEPS	RATIONALE
1. Sequence all course objectives in their order of emphasis and priority.	This provides the groundwork for the development of knowledge, skills, and attitudes. As the outline evolves, only *new* content elements are identified, as in a building process. Some of the most significant objectives frequently have the greatest amount of content elements.
2. Develop all the content elements in sequence.	All content elements should be reviewed to identify relationships, vacuums, and duplication.
3. Identify teaching methods separately.	This ensures that all content elements will be included in some teaching method. The specific content should be identified to give adequate direction to the student and faculty.
4. Select evaluative methods.	After all content elements and teaching methods are reviewed, the methods to be utilized to evaluate students for a grade will follow more easily and will have a greater degree of validity in terms of the ability of the student to meet the objectives to be measured.

Summary

The formative stage of the process consists of three components: curriculum design and requirements, level and course objectives, and content map. It is during this stage that the curriculum begins to take shape and gives the directive stage form and substance. The directive stage is used as a foundation upon which the curriculum plan is designed. The level and course objectives are identified based on the characteristics of the graduate and the content map is delineated based on the theoretical framework. The relationship of each component to the other and the relationship of the formative stage to the directive stage are shown throughout the chapter.

4

Functional Stage

The functional stage gives meaning and action to the entire curriculum process and has three components:

1. approaches to content
2. teaching methodology and learning experiences
3. validation of learning.

Within the functional stage, are reflected the day-to-day activities of a nursing program and from a student's perception it represents the total program of studies offered. Faculty and students identify most closely with the content being taught, the teaching approaches used, the experiences that facilitate learning, and the methods of evaluation used to validate such learning. Thus, if there are inconsistencies, difficulties will arise.

During this stage the faculty will identify what approaches to the content best reflects the curriculum that has been developed. It is inappropriate to pattern the content elements according to a particular textbook relating to the subject. Content can be offered in a variety of ways such as the study of diseases in a series, a human body systems model, a unified conceptual approach which emphasizes a particular theoretical framework such as adaptation, and any combination of the above. It is essential that the content approach not be decided in a simplistic manner but truly reflect the previous curriculum decisions about the content elements made by the faculty. Admittedly, this is a very difficult task but it is imperative if the directive and formative stages are to have any significance.

Teaching methods must not be assumed but selected to reflect the most appropriate way in which the content can be most easily learned. Learning experiences need to speak specifically to course objectives and need to integrate the content into every activity required of the student. The validation of learning through quantitative and qualitative measurements (formative evaluation) is an integral part of the functional stage and will be used to determine the success of the courses taught.

During this stage, continuous modification tends to occur since both the faculty and students are involved in a never-ending evaluation of each other and the program. Sometimes it is difficult to assess whether the components are appropriately and fully developed or whether a particular group of faculty and/or students are having difficulty accepting the curriculum. Since revisions frequently result as students and faculty change and often without careful consideration of their appropriateness to the developed philosophy, etc., the best developed curriculum will need a total review at least every three to four years. The depth and breadth of the modifications made within the courses will strongly influence the length of time a curriculum is functional. This need will become evident to the faculty when it realizes that the content being taught is not fully supportive of the philosophy or is not relevant to a new body of knowledge.

Approaches to Content

Within the last decade the most frequently used terms to describe a nursing curriculum are the "medical model" or "integrated model." Such terminology is offered as a way of explaining the faculty's perception of its approach to content in teaching nursing. The greater the faculty involvement in curriculum development, the more likely the faculty is to move toward the integrated model and away from the medical model. Since the meaning and/or significance of this movement is not clearly understood, little real changes in teaching become evident to the faculty and students.

There is no consensus among nurse educators on the characteristics of an integrated curriculum. And, for that reason, confusion persists as to whether or not it truly exists and to what extent within any given program it is implemented. In 1974 it was defined as "blending the nursing content in such a way that the 'parts' or 'specialties' are no longer distinguishable"[1] Implied in such a definition is that the melding of parts or specialities leads us to a whole, and that the medical specialties once meshed would give us nursing content. This definition does not truly define what integration is in terms of the discipline of nursing. An integrated nursing model in this sense is defined as a model which focuses on nursing as a practice discipline that has a strong foundation in nursing theories/concepts and their relationships which guide practice. Essential here are the following assumptions:

Nursing is a discipline separate and distinct from the natural and pure sciences.

Nursing education is distinctly different from medical education in its content and emphasis.

---

[1] Gertrude Torres, "Educational Trends and the Integrated Curriculum Approach in Nursing," in *Unifying the Curriculum—The Integrated Approach* (New York: NLN, 1974), p. 2.

Nursing as a practice profession needs to focus primarily on a process (the nursing, teaching, or communicative process).

Nursing knowledge is most useful when it supports a greater understanding through generalizations.

If we agree on the above assumptions, then an integrated nursing curriculum is one *that uses a process orientation as its approach to theoretical nursing knowledge which encourages generalizations.*

Table 4.1 explains the differences among models that are being used to implement the current philosophies of nursing programs. This movement from the traditional medical model to multiple nursing models is being enhanced by philosophical statements relating to human beings as being holistic and health as viewed on a continuum. These models should be viewed on a continuum and it must be realized that any curriculum model may incorporate aspects of another.

The traditional and semimedical models (I and II in Table 4.1), which do not support a conceptual holistic view, educate by approaching content as a series of specialties in a variety of patterns. For example, in the traditional medical model, nursing arts is usually followed by medical–surgical, then pediatrics, obstetrical, or psychiatric nursing, with public health nursing at the end of the program. The content approach is disease/illness oriented, and the environment within the hospital sets the stage for most clinical learning experiences, except public health nursing. The traditional medical model continues to be used by some, even though few philosophical statements and identified content elements would support its use. Implied is the belief that medical science as applied to the nursing process reflects the theory and practice of nursing. The semimedical model selects some common content appropriate for all the specialties and is often referred to as the "core." This frequently includes the content from generalizations that can be drawn among the specialties, for example, oxygenation, decompensation, and inflammation. The extent to which such core content is developed depends on the fac-

Table 4.1

Models of Nursing

PROPOSITION WITHIN THE PHILOSOPHY	CONTENT APPROACH	POTENTIAL CONTENT ELEMENTS
I—TRADITIONAL MEDICAL MODEL Nursing knowledge is primarily *based* on medical science and focuses on nursing specialties as its approach to practice.	Medical and nursing specialties	Pathophysiology and disease; Medical, surgical, obstetrical, pediatric, and psychiatric nursing
II—SEMIMEDICAL MODEL Nursing is *based* on both the specific knowledge within each medical specialty and those generalizations that can be drawn from them.	Core content plus medical and nursing specialties	Core concepts— Oxygenation Immobility Pain Medical model content elements
III—INTEGRATED MODEL Nursing is a process-oriented discipline which has as its focus the human beings' status on the health continuum and which is based on the knowledge derived from its discipline.	Nursing process Health status Health continuum Nursing theories/ concepts	Decision-making theories Leadership theories Levels of wellness theories Adaptation theories Self-care theories Interaction/transaction theories

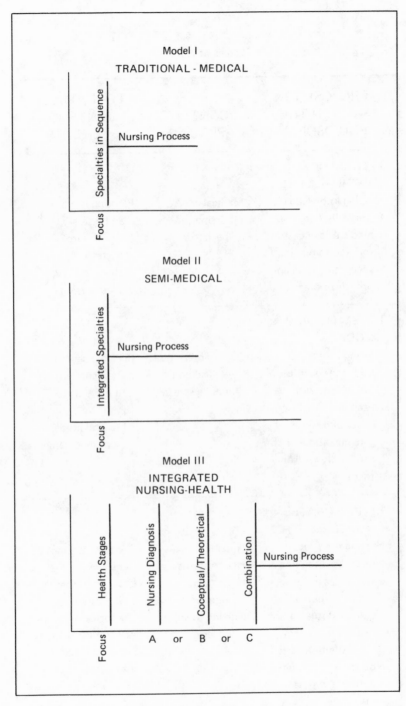

Figure 4.1
Models of Approaches to Content

ulty's ability to move away from the medical model and better conceptualize its views on nursing. In the semimedical model the core course may be followed by courses such as: Nursing of Adults, Nursing of Children, Community Health Nursing or Biophysiological Nursing of Adults and Children, Psycho/ Social Nursing of Children and Adults, Community Health Nursing, or courses labeled Nursing I, II, III, etc., focusing on developmental stages—all include a blending of concepts from medical–surgical nursing, pediatric nursing, psychiatric nursing, and so on.

The integrated nursing model (III in Table 4.1) supports a holistic view. It approaches content with a health or wellness orientation and focuses on the theories and concepts of nursing, integrating related theories, like decision making, which support or compliment the nursing theories. Course descriptions are derived from the theoretical framework such as: Use of the Nursing Process with Healthy Individuals.

In reviewing the models, it should be noted that the medical model reflects what is foundational or basic to nursing knowledge rather than accomplishing what the integrated model does, which is explain the discipline of nursing. The potential content elements within the integrated model tend to be much more theory oriented. Approaching nursing content without a disease orientation does have a profound effect on the curriculum.

Thus, it becomes even more obvious that the approach to teaching the content elements is strongly influenced by the directive and formative stages of the curriculum process. This approach to content in combination with course objectives is essentially the basis upon which the faculty develops the specific course content. Also, it is important to identify the criteria that are significant in the development of any course of study. The criteria include the following:

The depth and breadth of the content must be appropriate for the learner. As nursing increasingly identifies its body of knowledge through research, the selection of content will become even more difficult. The faculty, especially the members oriented toward the specialty areas, tends to want to offer a greater degree of depth than may be appropriate for the type of practitioner that is identified in the characteristics.

The validity of the content must be assessed. Nursing content must be taught in the framework of whether or not it has been empirically tested. Nursing theories/concepts which have not been validated through research should be offered in that context.

The content must reflect the emerging health care system and the changing role of the nurse. An educator must focus on providing the consumer of nursing care with a practitioner who will function for some 30 to 50 years.

Content which encourages generalizations should be emphasized. Since there is an ever-increasing body of knowledge, it is important to approach the selection of content in a way that provides for the greatest amount of learning.

The content must be progressive, starting with areas that are more easily learned and foundational to areas of content that are highly dependent on previous learning and require synthesis. This should *not* be viewed as going from the simple to the complex, but rather as an approach in which emphasis is placed on the learner's ability to deal with specific pieces of information at any given period time.

The content should motivate the student to learn. Properly sequenced content approaches will guide and direct the learner to want to pursue each area of knowledge more fully. It is not only how well the content is presented that is significant but also how such content relates to what the student perceives as essential in her or his learning.

The content must reflect the level within the cognitive, affective, and psychomotor domains that is appropriate in relation to the stated objectives. Whether we wish the student to achieve at a cognitive level of comprehension or at the level of synthesis strongly influences the approach to content that is appropriate for the learner.

There are difficulties encountered in identifying the appropriate content from the stated course objectives and theoretical framework. Some of these difficulties are listed below:

poorly developed components within the directive and deductive stages; content elements not clearly distinguishable;

lack of congruence between the faculty's graduate preparation and knowledge and the content that is being developed;

inadequate in-service education for faculty;

lack of adequate planning to provide time and resources for this activity when it is frequently viewed as the "end" of the curriculum development process.

A careful analysis should be made periodically to ensure that the content is progressive and appropriate. Since this activity is often delegated to the faculty members who teach the nursing course, communications systems within the program tend to weaken unless a content map or something similar is developed.

Teaching Methodology and Learning Experiences

Once the objectives and content elements have been developed, careful attention must be given to the identification of appropriate teaching methods. These methods include all those activities and learning experiences developed by the faculty with input from students that facilitate learning on the part of the student. Recognition also must be given to the fact that students' life experiences have an impact on their ability to meet the objectives.

Generally, little or no attention is given to teaching methodology and learning experiences by the curriculum committee since individual faculty members teaching the content usually decide what methods to use. All too frequently the methods and experiences selected are based on the faculty members' perception of their own ability to use various teaching methods instead of on the dictates of the objectives and content. Careful planning before the content is presented is vital and requires time on the part of the faculty.

The philosophy of the program in relation to those statements about learning has a strong impact on the methods used to teach. Usually, such statements help to clarify the roles of the student and the teacher in the learning process. An example of this can be found in Table 4.2.

Also, within the philosophy, direction can be seen that will guide the faculty in its selection of learning experiences. Propositions that relate to the emerging role of the nurse often give strong clues to which experiences would be most appropriate. If the faculty believes that the nurse will have a greater involvement in the care of healthy individuals in the future, and if the objectives were appropriately developed to reflect this belief, learning experiences should be identified that will assist the student to understand the criteria for health and to have clinical learning experiences with healthy clients. Frequently there is a contradiction between the faculty's belief about nursing's role in relation to the health status of clients and the clinical environments in which the students are taught. For example, the emphasis in course content is placed on health teaching to maintain the client's optimum level of wellness, but the student is sent to a hospital in-patient unit to achieve the related objective. A well-baby or adult screening clinic would be more appropriate. All too frequently, decisions are made to offer learning experiences in previously utilized and organized health care agencies such as hospitals and health departments without considering the many other health care facilities available such as schools, industry, and mobile health units.

Within each objective, the level of achievement and the depth and breadth of the content elements to be learned need to influence the teaching methods. Objectives which speak to knowledge or comprehension can often be achieved through

Table 4.2

Relationships Between Philosophy and Teaching Methods

PHILOSOPHICAL STATEMENT	APPROPRIATE TEACHING METHODS	
	Student's role	*Teacher's role*
The learner has responsibility for independence, self-direction	Develops own bibliography Identifies area of strengths and weaknesses in terms of meeting the objectives Seeks assistance when appropriate Assumes responsibility for learning Takes independent study course	Provides guidelines for developing bibliography Validates areas of strength and weaknesses Sets parameters for required learning experiences Provides criteria for meeting objectives
The educator assists students to learn through counseling, guiding, and challenging the student	Uses suggestions of teacher to increase learning Uses teacher-provided guidelines Asks questions, shares ideas	Counsels students in relation to their needs as learners Guides each learning activity Stimulates the student to think and question

the use of a lecture, an audio visual experience, or a programmed learning activity. Those which relate to synthesis or evaluation require methods that facilitate and challenge the students' thinking process such as independently developed position papers, panel discussions, debates, or seminar activities in small groups. The content also has to have a match with the approaches used to educate. Content elements, in the form of concepts/theories, can be offered to a large group by means of the lecture methods. Content which relates to values must clearly be offered in a nonthreatening small-group environment in which the focus is on discussion and analysis. Skills, whether they are technical, intellectual, or communicative, need to be taught in a variety of ways that support reinforcement because skills require continued practice. This can be accomplished through video taping interviews, process recording techniques, practice laboratory experiences, or by caring for clients in the clinical settings.

Learning experiences that assist the student in meeting the objectives must be viewed in their totality rather than as isolated situations. Classroom experiences must relate to skills and attitudes and laboratory experiences must expand and reinforce the knowledge achieved within the classroom environment. Table 4.3 reflects the recognition of such relationships.

Thus, multiple learning experiences are usually essential to meet any particular objective. Similarly, one learning experience can assist the student in meeting more than one objective. However, both the faculty and the students often find it difficult to specify which objectives match which learning experiences. Faculty and students need to understand the essential rationale for each learning experience. Thus, prior to each learning experience, whether it be within the classroom or client care situation, the major objective(s) of the experience should be discussed.

The resources, especially in terms of the time and energy the faculty and students need to achieve the objectives, must be an integral part of the selection of learning experiences. Faculty and students need to be reasonable in their expectations of each other and they must mutually interact in relation

Table 4.3

Relationship Between Classroom and Clinical Experiences

OBJECTIVE	CONTENT ELEMENTS	LEARNING EXPERIENCES
Identifies the ethical and legal responsibility of the nurse using the nursing process	Knowledge of ethical and legal responsibilities of the nurse Skill in applying such knowledge when using the nursing process Attitude reflecting responsibility for legal and ethical knowledge	Provides classroom discussion and readings on ethical and legal issues Implementation of nursing care reflective of knowledge of ethical/legal issues Approach to client that demonstrates ethical concern and legal responsibility

to the value of each learning experience and the time and energy expended. For example, the faculty should not require students to read an extensive list of references which are duplicative or poorly developed in terms of the objectives that are to be achieved. Term papers should only be required that are essential to the learning activity and essential to meet the objective(s). Term papers should be limited in their length so that only the essential ideas are presented by the students and so that the faculty can devote an adequate amount of time to review them. Clinical laboratory hours should be limited to the amount of time essential to meet the objectives rather than to meet some traditional predetermined schedule. In limiting the use of resources, both the faculty and student can better focus their energies on what has to be accomplished and both teaching and learning can become more exciting.

Since students differ in their abilities to learn and their previous experiences, multiple learning activities, with options whenever possible, should be offered. For example, students who function best and are most comfortable in group activities may learn more effectively in assignments that facilitate group interaction; other students may find it easier to meet the same objectives through individually oriented experiences. The faculty must focus on the ability of the student to meet the objective, not on how the particular objective is to be met. Meeting individualized needs tends to demand a greater degree of flexibility and is more time-consuming on the part of the faculty but essential if at all possible. Careful assessment of the students' learning styles and the faculty's trust in the students' ability to identify those experiences which best assist them in learning are important.

The environment in which the students' learning activities occur can have a profound impact on their ability to meet the objectives. This is especially true in clinical laboratory experiences since these experiences tend to be stressful and anxiety provoking. Support systems need to be developed that allow learning to take place. Examples would be group discussions that offer both faculty and peer support and appropriate feedback if difficulties arise. Realistic expectations also need to be identified within any given environment since some are more supportive than others and offer differing opportunities to learn at any given period of time.

Other variables that affect the selection of teaching methods are the ratio of students to faculty, the availability of teaching aids, and the ability of the faculty to use any given method. The teaching methods to be used by the faculty must be identified prior to the teaching of a course in the context of the teaching methods' advantages and limitations. An outline is presented in Table 4.4.

The method the faculty selects may be of greater significance to the learning process than any other variable. Preparation of the content must relate to the methods that will facilitate learning. Students should be informed prior to class activities so that they can be better prepared to participate in their own

Table 4.4

Advantages and Limitations of Teaching Methods

TEACHING METHODS	MAJOR ADVANTAGES	USUAL LIMITATIONS
Classroom activity (lecture) role-playing, etc. large group activity:	Provides the basic structure to guide learning	Tends not to focus on individual learning styles Supports a greater passivity on the part of the student Most economical in terms of use of space and faculty time
Small group activity	Allows for greater interactions between faculty and students as well as between students. Facilitates discussion of attitudes Allows for a greater degree of activity on the part of the student	Not as economical in terms of the use of time and space Faculty are often unprepared to work with small groups
Independent activities (term papers, readings, etc.)	Provides for reinforcement and greater clarity of previous learning on an individual basis	Often lacks adequate faculty guidance to achieve optimum learning Since it is less directive in terms of learning, can

Table 4.4

Advantages and Limitations of Teaching Methods (*continued*)

TEACHING METHODS	MAJOR ADVANTAGES	USUAL LIMITATIONS
		cause duplication or vacuums in the content elements Economical in terms of space but takes up faculty time
Laboratory experiences (school, clinical settings, etc.)	Reinforces knowledge and attitudes while allowing students to practice the psychomotor skills Provides a "real" world view of nursing Allows for the use of role models as a learning strategy Most supportive of the concept that faculty members are catalysts in the learning activity	Difficult to control the variables that influence learning Requires the greatest amount of time and energy on the part of the faculty and the students Most costly learning activity

learning. Some teaching methods vary in their demand for outside readings prior to class. For example, a small group activity focusing on a social issue in which readings are required would expect a different preparation on the part of the student than would the demonstration of a new technical skill. The student needs to know whether she or he will be expected to actively participate, as through discussion, or whether the lecture method, which supports a more passive role on the part of the student, will be utilized.

The problems most often expressed by students pertain to the teaching method that the faculty uses. The consistent use of lectures as a method of presentation tends to have a nonchallenging effect on the student and supports her or his concept that learning occurs by listening and repetition. Students view faculty members as the givers of knowledge and themselves as the receivers. Students do not see themselves as accountable for learning. Also, repeatedly using modules for learning can give students the idea that independent activities such as responding to written questions rather than to faculty and peers facilitate learning. There must be balance between totally faculty-oriented approaches in which the student is dependent and totally student-oriented approaches in which the student is independent as a learner. Interdependent activities which actively involve both the teacher and the learner need to be emphasized. Thus, whenever feasible, a variety of teaching methods should be used. This is especially important since students are heterogenous in their learning approaches.

The roles of faculty and students within the clinical settings need to be carefully identified if client/patient-oriented activities are to facilitate learning. To a beginning student of nursing, this represents a break from the traditional lecture or seminar approach to education and it is also substantially different from the approaches used in chemistry or other laboratories. Human interactions, assuming responsibility for others' welfare, and a greater degree of independent activities are required within a generally stressful environment which has as its major goal the care of people rather than the teaching of students. This requires that the learner have a clear understanding of what the faculty expects and what her or his role is within the clinical environment. The following emphasizes the roles the faculty and student must play as well as their reciprocal roles:

FACULTY	STUDENT	RECIPROCAL
Identify appropriate environment for particular learning activity	Orient self to the environment as much as possible	Evaluate the laboratory experience as an environment for learning
Select client/patient within each setting	Offer input into the type of clients that would enhance learning	Interact to achieve optimum nursing care for the client/patient
Inform the student prior to the experience of the obtives to be achieved.	Have adequate preparation for the laboratory experience	Discuss and clarify the purpose of each experience
Facilitate learning through consistent feedback	Provide input regarding the progress of the learning experience	Interact in a mutually enhancing way to facilitate each other's activity
Provide an adequate amount of time to allow student to achieve objective	Utilize the available time to achieve optimum learning	Evaluate the frequency and amount of time needed for the clinical experience
Evaluate student activities for learning	Evaluate own activities in terms of meeting the objective	Share evaluation to facilitate further learning
Assume responsibility as an educator for guiding and facilitating learning	Be responsible for one's own learning and the results of the clinical activity	Accept responsibility for the outcome of experience

Validation of Learning

In any educational process it is essential that some mechanism be developed to validate learning in relation to the behavioral objectives. Such mechanisms usually take the form of measurement tools which tend to be quantitative rather than qualitative. Admittedly, qualitative data primarily reflect a professional judgment approach which strongly influences the development of quantitatively developed tools. Thus, evaluation can be defined as a systematic process of gathering data through the use of primarily quantitative tools to validate the student's achievement in relation to the content elements (knowledge, skills, and attitudes) within the stated objectives. This is a form of *criterion-referenced* evaluation since it is based on the student's achievement as related to the behavioral objectives rather than *norm-referenced* which compares students to others at a similar level as done with NLN achievement tests.

There are *three* types of evaluation that occur within a program which involve the students' ability to achieve the stated objectives. These are:

1. evaluation for continued learning

2. evaluation for grading

3. evaluation for curriculum revision

The latter will be discussed in a later chapter under curriculum evaluation. Although any evaluation of the students offers data that could be used by all three types, it is essential that the faculty conceptualizes and develops them differently. For example, final examinations are developed to assess learning for grading purposes and should *not* be viewed as a learning activity. Admittedly, learning frequently does occur, but it is not the major purpose. Similarly, ongoing evaluation in the clinical area to enhance further learning should not be graded since the evaluation may interfere with the learning process. The major differences between evaluation for learning and grading are identified as follows:

LEARNING	GRADING
Provides for *continuous* assessment of students' achievement and enhances the concept of progressive learning	Provides for *periodic* assessment of students' achievement to support progression in the program
Based mostly on *informally* developed *qualitative* methods	Based mostly on formally planned *qualitative* methods
Facilitates *individuality* and *creativity*	Supports *group* orientation and *conformity*
Provides *nondocumented* data	Provides *documented* data to validate teacher decisions on evaluation
Is oriented to *teacher-student* interactions for assessment data	*Teacher* developed assessment tool
Provides for *immediate* feedback relating to a *limited* learning experience	Provides for *long-range* feedback relating to *multiple* learning experiences
More clinically oriented process	Greater *knowledge* focused process

For the most part, evaluation for learning has a greater commitment to continuous, individualized, and informal data collection, while evaluation for grading focuses on periodic, group, and formal assessment. Realistically, the dichotomy between the two may be more theoretical than actual within the learning environment. For example, immediate feedback may be possible after a final exam. This sometimes provides students with data to better understand their individual needs for learning, but it is impractical and is not the purpose of a final examination. It is best to separate evaluation for learning from evaluation for grading to give the faculty and students a greater sense of purpose and clarity in relation to the whole concept of evaluation. This should lessen the conflict and frustration caused by the confusion as to why certain evaluation methods are used.

Certain assumptions need to be accepted in relation to evaluation of students for continued learning and for grading.

1. Valid evaluation methods are essential if educators are to be accountable.

   Since educators are accountable for assuring the public that the characteristics of the graduate are achieved, it is important that the evaluation of students during each phase of the program be based on valid and reliable tools. Also, the students have a right to be appropriately evaluated since they have a large investment in their educational pursuits.

2. The faculty has the responsibility to develop those tools which will be used to assess the student's achievement in relation to the developed objective(s).

   Tools developed by outside agencies which do not clearly relate to the objectives are inappropriate. Such tools as NLN achievement tests and state board examinations should *not* be used to evaluate the student for learning or grading unless the faculty can specifically validate that the knowledge skills and attitudes they measure are within the behavioral objectives. Since such tools are not developed within the context of the developed curriculum, it should be assumed that they are not useful.

3. Evaluation forms and measurement tools are basically more subjective than objective and require continued reassessment in terms of their ability to measure the student's achievement.

The development of any evaluation mechanism, including a measurement tool, is based on the qualitative judgment of the educator. Decisions on the methods, tools, and specific content elements to emphasize within any measurement tool are subjective. Some are viewed as more objective than others since they provide for a more defined criteria for measurement and grading. Multiple choice questions would be an example. Others in which the results are difficult to assess are viewed as more subjective. Term papers would be an example. Yet, in the development of any tool, some subjectivity on the part of the educator must be recognized and accepted.

The selection of specific evaluation tools should be done within the context of the tools' ability to assess the expected behaviors within the course objective. Table 4.5 identifies the major considerations that should be used in selecting such tools. The list of tools reflects those most commonly used and should not be viewed as all inclusive. Some written tests offer the most objective criteria for grading; therefore, this form of evaluation should be used unless either the level of achievement or the content elements can best be measured in another way. For example, clinical evaluation is the most time-consuming to plan and the most difficult to develop specific criteria for grading purposes since it is almost impossible to control the environmental variables. Yet, it is the only method available to truly evaluate the students' ability to assess an individual and implement specific care. Similarly, measuring the learners' ability to conceptualize or find new relationships can better be achieved through independent activities rather than through written examinations.

Assessment of Curriculum Process

When the curriculum is completed, it must be assessed as a total package to ensure consistency among its component parts. Crucial to the activity is the validation that every learning experience reflects the decisions made by the faculty. All the time and effort that is expended is of *no* significance if the

Table 4.5

Major Considerations in the Use of Evaluation Tools

EVALUATION TOOLS	MAJOR CONSIDERATIONS FOR USE
Written test— Objective questions in written examination	Provides the most objective criteria for grading Requires time and effort to develop an appropriate grid as well as mea- sure validity and reliability Useful in measuring knowledge, com- prehension, and application. Cannot measure synthesis
Essay test— Response to written statements	Requires less time to prepare Difficult to establish specific objec- tive criteria for grading Allows student a greater degree of creativity in responding Measures more generalized than spe- cific knowledge Useful in measuring analysis and synthesis Limited in scope of knowledge to be measured
Simulation— Responses to audio- visual experience such as a film	Time consuming and expensive to develop by faculty Difficult to identify if outside re- sources used Difficult to establish specific criteria for grading Measures knowledge and attitudes as well as such skills as critical think- ing and analysis

Table 4.5

Major Considerations in the Use of Evaluation Tools (*continued*)

EVALUATION TOOLS	MAJOR CONSIDERATIONS FOR USE
Independent activity— Term papers	Most often very time consuming for students and faculty Difficult to establish specific criteria for grading Can measure knowledge, skills, and attitudes but is more useful in the areas of conceptualizing or integrating knowledge and in measuring analysis and synthesis
Clinical performance test—	Time consuming in terms of planning and grading Difficult to develop specific criteria for grading Almost impossible to control the variables within the clinical environment that affect evaluation Most appropriate method to assess the students' ability to implement care. Must use observation and questioning to validate observations. Should not be used to measure areas that can be assessed by other evaluative tools

learner does not feel the impact. All too often, the content elements taught on a day-to-day basis show little relationship to the philosophy or theoretical framework. Thus, the teacher needs to be able to critique the finished product and continuously monitor each component to strengthen its impact on the learning process. Curriculum development is a never-ending process of refinement.

The criteria for the assessment of the curriculum process to ensure consistency among its component parts are as follows:

1. The flow of the content elements can be seen within all the components, especially between the philosophy and learning experiences.

    Example: Within the philosophy, society may be viewed as influenced by cultural norms. Sequentially, anthropology should be a required course, and the learner should assess the client and/or family in the context of his or her cultural norms. Also, texts used by the learner need to support this emphasis.

2. The terms used may have a variety of meanings within the discipline but they must be consistent in their meaning within the specific program.

    Example: The nursing process may have been identified within the philosophy as including the nursing diagnosis as one of its components. Within the glossary of terms, the definition of nursing diagnosis must be clear so that members of the faculty do not cause confusion among themselves and for the learner. Each component within the curriculum must use the term in a similar manner which supports the definition.

3. The ideas expressed among and within each component are supportive rather than contradictory.

    Example: The philosophy may emphasize humans as holistic and the role of the nurse as one who promotes health. To be consistent, learning activities must focus on client health in a holistic manner rather than experiences which emphasize the medically oriented biological approach to illness prevention. Health promotion such as teaching nutritional needs to the client is different from providing for immunization in a newborn clinic, which is disease prevention. Also, written examinations should validate the learner's ability to relate to the holistic concept.

At this point, the curriculum should be fully operative. Faculty and students should be familiar with all of the components and should be able to monitor what is happening, make minor revisions, and enjoy the fruits of their labor.

Summary

The functional stage of the curriculum process consists of three components: approaches to content, teaching methodology and learning experiences, and validation of learning. This stage shows the curriculum in action and is generally most visible to faculty and students. The medical model, semimedical model, and integrated nursing model are discussed as approaches to content. The faculty's beliefs about learning are used as the basis for discussing teaching and learning and the advantages and limitations of different teaching methods are delineated. Validation of learning is considered and the distinction between evaluation for learning and evaluation for grading is made.

5

Evaluative Stage

Comprehensive systematic curriculum evaluation is possible only at the time the curriculum is fully developed and implemented. While it must begin with the admission of first-year students, it cannot be fully realized until graduates of the program are out practicing since the object of curriculum evaluation is *to validate that the curriculum does what we say it will do in relation to the characteristics of the graduate.*

This is an excellent example of summative evaluation, the type of evaluation that takes place at the end of a program and gives a summary of what has been accomplished based on outcome characteristics, as opposed to formative evaluation that takes place at intervals during a course or program and shows the level of progress toward a given point.

The evaluative stage of the curriculum process places emphasis on evaluation of the curriculum rather than on faculty or student evaluation per se. It focuses on the *mean* achievements of students in relation to meeting level and course objectives and characteristics of the graduate. Students and faculty are integral parts of the process, but they are not the focus of the process. Also, curriculum evaluation does not interfere with the ongoing evaluation of students and faculty (formative and summative), which is an integral part of the education system. Curriculum evaluation uses the data collected at various points during the program as part of a systematic process.

The evaluative stage of the curriculum process consists of three components:

1. input
2. throughput
3. output

Input refers to what students bring to the educational environment. It is a combination of heredity, cultural background; previous learning experiences, motivation, attitudes, interest, knowledge, and skills. While it is impossible to know and use all of the input that students bring, it is useful for curriculum evaluation to know what students bring in relation to specific areas of the objectives, e.g., critical thinking, leadership skills, perception of professional nursing, assessment ability.

Throughput refers to the selected educational activities experienced by students as they progress through a particular educational program. End-of-course grades, level examinations, and comprehensive examinations are examples of the tools used to evaluate students' progression through a program.

Output refers to the level or degree of ability graduates of a particular program have in achieving the characteristics of the graduate in effect at the time of their graduation.

It must be remembered that for the purpose of curriculum evaluation all data used are in aggregate form (see Fig. 5.1).

The Input Component

The input component is most often the least used component of curriculum evaluation. This may be due to a certain skepticism on the part of the faculty or the lack of available adequate

A Quantitive Process

Input —— Throughout —— Output

Characteristics of Graduate

	Initial Evaluation	Intermediate Evaluation	Longitudinal Evaluation
Assessment	Diagnostic Preadmission and Preclinical Evaluation Tools	Level Comprehensive Tools	Comprehensive Tools at Termination of Program Followed by Longitudinal Studies
Analysis	Identification of Levels of Achievement of Prenursing Population (Mean Scores)	Achievement of Student Population of Behavioral Level Objectives (Mean Scores)	Identification of Level of Success of Graduate Population (Mean Scores)
Implications	Modification of Admission Criteria	Revision of Level Objectives and Learning Experiences	Modification and Redevelopment of Curriculum. Planning Continuing Education Programs for Alumnae
Evaluative Format	Formative	Formative	Summative

Figure 5.1

Design for Systematic Curriculum Evaluation Model

103

tools. However, the faculty should look at the characteristics of the graduate and select the three or four most relevant areas that can be pretested and would be important to validate at the end of the program. Although input can be used as a diagnostic tool to help students to succeed in the program, in curriculum evaluation it is used as a method of looking at what the students bring and the changes that may occur as the result of the educational program. This is the initial part of curriculum evaluation (see Initial Evaluation in Fig. 5.1). The faculty assesses the students in terms of what they bring—previous knowledge, attitudes, and skills—to the nursing program.

It is possible to use standardized tests related to mathematical skills, problem solving, leadership potential, assertiveness skills, and word associations that could have a bearing on the use of the nursing process or understanding research or selected leadership skills. The faculty needs to be selective in its use of any tests and should limit their use to those that are related to the philosophy, theoretical framework, and/or characteristics of the graduate of the program. There is no point in giving a pretest about leadership potential if leadership is not part of the program.

The faculty should remember that pretests are used to test the curriculum not the students in the program and as such should not be used in any way to penalize students with regard to progression in the program. This must be fully understood by administration, faculty, and students. However, it is possible to use the results of pretests to influence policy changes for subsequent groups of students.

The Throughput Component

The throughput component consists of all those activities in the educational program related to the functional stage of the curriculum process: teaching, learning, and grading. Throughput refers, in a literal sense, to what students go through in order to acquire the knowledge, attitudes, and skills to meet the characteristics of the graduate. Throughput takes into account cognitive, affective, and psychomotor learning.

The throughput component is the one most frequently used by the faculty; in fact, in many instances it is the only method used in evaluating the curriculum. The faculty is generally familiar with formative evaluation methods, the kind of evaluation that takes place at various intervals during a course or program. A level examination is an example of formative evaluation. Usually the faculty is able to improve the program based on formative evaluation feedback.

The faculty is constantly evaluating pieces of the curriculum and making decisions based on immediate feedback. All of the data collected as a result of formative evaluation are reviewed in terms of their possible impact or output. The throughput component can be viewed as the intermediate part of curriculum evaluation (see Intermediate Evaluation in Fig. 5.1). End-of-course evaluations and/or level evaluations to see how students meet course or level objectives can be viewed by faculty as summative evaluations for the end point of a course or sequence of courses (level). But for purposes of curriculum evaluation, since they occur at intervals, they are viewed as formative evaluation methods leading to the achievement of the characteristics of the graduate, which is an end point.

The Output Component

The output component looks at the graduate of the program in terms of the characteristics of the graduate as identified by the faculty. How well did the curriculum design achieve its purpose? This includes identifying those factors that inhibit and enhance meeting the characteristics of the graduate as well as longitudinal studies to look at the performance of graduates relative to the characteristics. For purposes of curriculum evaluation, graduates of a program should only be looked at in terms of the characteristics of the graduate that were operational at the time they graduated. But graduates can also be looked at in terms of current characteristics so that the faculty can plan for appropriate continuing education programs for alumnae to update their knowledge, skills, and attitudes. Generally, there are gradual but, in the main, minor changes in the characteristics of the graduate over a five-year period. As time progresses past the five-year period, major changes become more evident. One characteristic of the graduate that is generally present over the years and is relatively easy to assess is the graduates' involvement in life-long learning. The output component takes the long view: it is the longitudinal part of curriculum evaluation (see Longitudinal Evaluation in Fig. 5.1).

Figure 5.1 proposes a design for a systematic curriculum evaluation model in which the faculty assesses how well the students are doing and looks at where they are before they can move to the next step in the educational process. The faculty also analyzes the findings. The faculty looks at test or questionnaire results or other aggregate data which give indications of the students' and/or graduates' achievements or their perceptions of their achievements. Finally, the faculty decides what implications the findings have in relation to revision or modification of the curriculum. The model also provides the faculty with a measure of the validity of what the curriculum accomplished.

Summary

The evaluative and last stage of the curriculum process consists of three components: input, throughput, and output. Input deals with what the students bring with them, especially as related to specific items expressed in the characteristics of the graduates, such as leadership. Throughput refers to those educational activities the students participate in in order to meet the characteristics of the graduate. Output refers to the graduates of the program in relation to those characteristics operational at the time of their graduation.

Curriculum evaluation deals with the curriculum as a whole and determines how well the curriculum achieved its purpose. Are the graduates of the program able to meet the characteristics of the graduate as specified? Aggregate data are used to answer this question.

6

The Curriculum
Process:
An Assessment

In order to assess consistency among the components in terms of the criteria, a sample curriculum* will be outlined. This presentation is used to review the curriculum package from a process orientation rather than from a content orientation. It is offered to the readers as an exercise to facilitate their understanding of the curriculum process and as an example of the methodology that could be used to assess their own curriculum in terms of consistency. It does not reflect the ideal curriculum. Although a four-year nursing curriculum is presented, the process is similar when other types of educational programs are being assessed.

The following curriculum ideas for a Bachelor of Science in Nursing were developed at a state-supported university in a midwestern metropolitan area.

---

*The ideas for this sample curriculum were taken from the self-study report prepared by the faculty of Wright State University School of Nursing for NLN accreditation purposes, Fall, 1979. Faculty permission was granted for inclusion of these materials.

The philosophy of the sample curriculum is as follows:

The University
School of Nursing
PHILOSOPHY

The School of Nursing supports the University's purposes relating to teaching, research, and service. The faculty believes in the acquisition of knowledge from the past and present, as well as exploration of new knowledges, in the advancement of lifelong learning, the search for basic truth, and in the commitment of the University to the solution of problems affecting the larger community.

Human existence involves behavioral patterns, constant change, and interaction with biological, psychological, social, spiritual, and other forces in the environment. Although human existence contains elements of similarity, each person is the product of a unique genetic heritage in continuous and dynamic interaction with unique life experiences. Humanity is viewed in terms of ability to act and react in relation to a continuous process of change resulting in increasing complexity. Each individual functions within a set of values with the potential to be a thinking, creative, dignified, rational being.

Society within the human environment is composed of individuals, families, groups, and communities sharing a variety of common goals and values which change as the interests and needs of the members change. Social change evolves through the mutuality of relationships and the interaction of political and social forces which affect the individual's rights, responsibilities, and obligations. These dynamic forces determine the values and expectations placed upon the health care system as an integral part of society. The individual's interaction with the health care system is a reciprocal experience.

Health is the dynamic pattern of functioning whereby there is continued interaction with internal and external forces in an attempt to achieve the goal of maximum health potential. Health is influenced by inherent capabilities, growth and development, cultural background and totality of perception. Human dignity and the quality of life are influenced by the degree of vulnerability to health impairments and depletions. The availability of a variety of resources will influence health and serve to decrease vulnerability.

The practice of professional nursing is humanitarian in nature and requires a knowledge base in nursing. The integration of scientific, humanistic, and nursing concepts and theories, attainable through research, gives direction to this practice. The nursing process is interpersonal and caring in nature. In its totality, it includes assessment, diagnosis, planning, implementation, and evaluation, and it is the essence of professional practice. The nursing process is utilized with individuals and groups to maximize their potential for health.

The emerging role of the nurse practitioner involves a greater amount of independence in practice and an increasing accountability to the consumer of health and nursing care. This can be achieved through individualized care given on a continuous basis over an extended period of time. The professional nurse will increasingly be viewed as the nucleus of the health care system, as well as an advocate for the consumer. Through leadership and interaction skills, the nurse will act in consortium with the client and other health and nursing practitioners for health promotion and maintenance.

The baccalaureate program in nursing prepares a self-directed practitioner with a breadth of knowledge in nursing who functions as a generalist in a variety of health care settings. This practitioner is capable of functioning as a leader and as an initiator of change in the care-giving situation; supporting change within the health care system; coordinating and collaborating with consumers and inter-disciplinary health team members; utilizing selected theories, concepts, and research findings. Experiences are provided to help students define their role and develop personal and professional values and clinical competencies. This baccalaureate program provides the base for the master's preparation in nursing.

Learning is a dynamic lifetime growth process of behavioral changes which involve the development of maximum potential through a spirit of inquiry and self-motivation. Learning is a sequential process and combines cognitive, affective, and psychomotor components. The learner has responsibility for independence, self-direction, and reaching a level of self-realization. The educator has responsibility for determining and implementing quality education which is accomplished through sharing, counseling, guiding, and challenging. The educator and learner in nursing must continually evolve a greater understanding of the relationships among theory, research, and practice. This understanding facilitates the development of nursing theory and practice, provides a climate conducive to intellectual pursuits, contributes productively toward the higher standards of teaching, and encourages independent thought and creative endeavors.

Table 6.1 shows the direct relationship between the philosophy and the theoretical framework. Propositions relating to the key concepts are used as the basis for the identification of specific content elements which also provide structure through strands. Note the relationships among the propositions, content elements, theories, and structure in Table 6.2. These relationships support the significance and need for a well-developed set of propositions which in totality reflects the philosophy of the program. The content elements identified are theories that provide the learners with the necessary content to truly comprehend the meaning of the propositions. Professional judgments are required to expand the content elements even though at times they are not specifically mentioned in the propositional statements. For example, the health care

Table 6.1

A Theoretical Framework from Philosophical Base

CONCEPTS	HUMANITY	SOCIETY	HEALTH	NURSING
Philosophy	Human existence involves *behavioral* patterns, constant *change* and *interaction* with *biological, psychological, social, spiritual,* and other forces in the *environment.* Although human existence contains elements of similarity, each person is the product of a unique *genetic* heritage in continuous and dynamic *interaction* with unique life experiences. Humanity is viewed in terms of ability to act and react in relation to a continuous process of *change* resulting in increasing complexity. Each individual functions within a set of *values*	Society within the human environment is composed of *individuals, families, groups,* and *communities* sharing a variety of common goals and values which change as the interest and *needs* of the members change. Social change evolves through the mutuality of relationships and the interaction of *political* and *social* forces which affect the individual's rights, responsibilities, and obligations. These dynamic forces determine the *values* and expectations placed upon the health care *system* as an integral part of society. Individual's in-	Health is the dynamic *pattern* of functioning, whereby there is continued interaction with internal and external forces in an attempt to achieve the goal of maximum health potential. Health is influenced by *inherent capabilities, growth and development, culture,* and *totality of perception.* Human dignity and the quality of life are influenced by the degree of *vulnerability* to health impairments and depletions. The availability of a variety of resources will influence health and serve to decrease vulnerability.	The practice of professional nursing is humanitarian in nature and requires a knowledge base in nursing. The integration of *scientific, humanistic,* and *nursing concepts and theories,* attainable through research, gives direction to this practice. The nursing process is *interpersonal* and caring in nature. In its totality, it includes *assessment, diagnosis, planning, implementation,* and *evaluation,* and is the essence of professional practice. The nursing process is utilized with individuals and groups to maximize their potential for health. The emerging role of the nurse practitioner involves a greater amount of independence in

Table 6.1

A Theoretical Framework from Philosophical Base *(continued)*

CONCEPTS	HUMANITY	SOCIETY	HEALTH	NURSING
	with the potential to be a thinking, creative, dignified, rational being.	teraction with the health care system is a reciprocal experience.		practice and an increasing *accountability* to the consumer of health and nursing care. This can be achieved through individualized care given on a continuous basis over an extended period of time. The professional nurse will increasingly be viewed as the *nucleus* of the health care system, as well as an *advocate* for the consumer. Through *leadership* and interaction skills, the nurse will act in consortium with the client and other health and nursing practitioners for health promotion and maintenance.

Content Elements:	Additional Content Elements:	Additional Content Elements:	Additional Content Elements:
Knowledge— Biology, Psychology, Sociology, Religion/Philosophy	*Knowledge*—Political Science, health care system	*Knowledge*—Human health patterns and available resources	*Knowledge*—Nursing, research
Theories— Change, value, interaction, behavioral, social, environmental, communication, humanistic, genetic, personality	*Theories*—Family, group, political systems, need, organizational	*Theories*—Developmental cultural, health–stress, crisis, wellness, epidemiological	*Theories*—Nursing, interpersonal evaluation, learning, leadership, conflict, decision making, role
Skills— Identify unique pattern	*Skills*—Can interact with a changing society	*Skills*—Utilize resources; reduce vulnerability	*Skills*—Nursing process and its components
Attitudes— Value human dignity; accept impact of environmental forces	*Attitudes*—Support societies, common goals, and values; individuals have rights, responsibilities, and obligations	*Attitudes*—Health as a value	*Attitudes*—Supports independence, consumer advocacy, and individualized care
Structure: (Strands)			
Vertical— Human existence	*Vertical*—Society Health care systems	*Vertical*—Health states *Horizontal*—Health prevention patterns; health promotion and maintenance	*Vertical*—Research, leadership *Horizontal*—Nursing process, accountability and responsibility, interdependent-independent functions

Table 6.2

Relationships of Components in Directive Stage

PROPOSITIONS	CONTENT ELEMENTS— THEORIES	STRUCTURE
Human existence involves behavioral patterns, constant *change* and *inter- action*	Change and interactive theories	Human existence
Individual's inter- action with the health care *system* is a reciprocal experience	Systems and organiza- tional theories	Society Health care system
Health is influenced by inherent capa- bilities, *growth* and *development, cul- ture*	Developmental, cul- tural theories	Health status Health care system
The nursing process is interpersonal in nature	Interpersonal theory Peplau's concept of nursing	Nursing process

system mentioned in the proposition requires the learner to understand not only systems theory but also organizational theory. Thus, it is added as a necessary dimension. Similarly, in the theoretical framework the major theories are identified within the area of health such as stress and crisis even though they are not spelled out in the propositions. Since such ex- tensions are almost limitless, it is essential that only those areas that have a strong relationship to the propositions be identified.

Figure 6.1 identifies the strands supporting the theoretical framework. Content strands are vertical and relate to all key concepts. Process strands are horizontal and only relate to health and nursing. Since the nursing process is utilized to recognize health potential and promote health, it is a constant activity and is viewed as the "art of the discipline" requiring continued practice. As a matter of fact, all horizontal strands are both content and process. The learner initially learns the process which appears as content. In other words, process is content, but content is not usually process. Thus, the educator's perception of what is content and what is process plays a strong role in how the strands will be developed. Such decisions offer guidelines for implementation of the curriculum and a total commitment on the part of the faculty.

It should be carefully noted that each strand is further developed to give detail and greater clarity for the later development of level objectives and the content map. The glossary of terms can be instrumental here. For example, leadership, a vertical strand, provides the content necessary for students to learn to coordinate care in the third year and to facilitate collaboration in the fourth year. Research, another vertical strand, initially guides the student in understanding research so that during the fourth year the learner will use research for practice and for assisting in gathering data.

The horizontal and vertical strands of the theoretical framework provide guidance for the development of level and course objectives and the content map. The vertical strands of the conceptual framework support the concept of progressive learning and are content oriented. The horizontal strands are process oriented and are consistently reinforced throughout the program. The two types of strands are described as follows:

Vertical Strands

Health Continuum. This emphasizes the client's health status and potential as viewed on a continuum. Primarily,

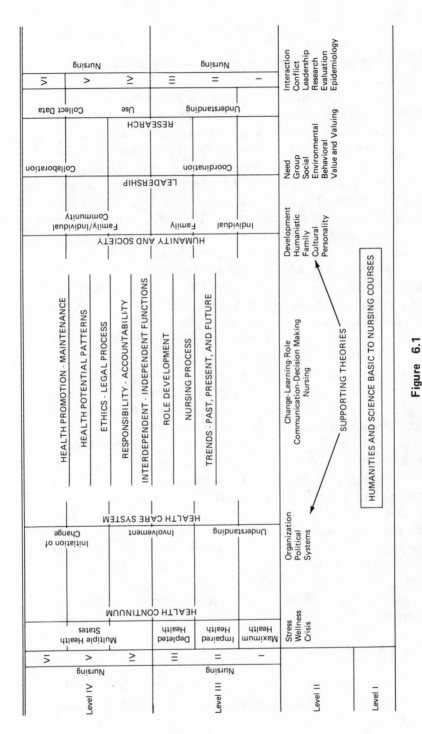

Figure 6.1

Curriculum Strands Supporting Theoretical Framework

118

the emphasis is on health and an in-depth understanding of the client's health status followed by an increasing emphasis of health potential. Thus, it is viewed as a vertical strand demonstrating progressive learning and approaching previous concepts and/or theories in relation to differing states of health.

Health Care System. Students initially are exposed to the present health care system. Progressing through the curriculum, students are expected to increase their leadership involvement as the nucleus of the system and identify ways in which they can assist planned change to better meet the health and nursing needs of the consumers.

Leadership. One way this is viewed is through the activities of coordination, collaboration, and consultation. Emphasis is placed on the interactive and nursing processes utilizing leadership theories to provide quality nursing care.

Research. This strand is introduced early in the nursing curriculum in terms of an appreciation and understanding of the need for nursing research. This is later followed by utilizing research, and gathering data.

Humanity and Society. This strand consists of individuals, families, communities, and vulnerable groups. The focus of the client population progresses from individuals to communities.

Horizontal Strands

Nursing Process. This is viewed as a horizontal strand since, in its totality, it represents the essence of the practice of nursing and is a deliberate, intellectual approach. An in-depth understanding is expected of the student early at the junior level of the nursing curriculum. Increasing breadth is accomplished through the utilization of the nursing process throughout the upper division.

Responsibility and Accountability. Since these concepts are considered an integral part of all learning experiences and an essential characteristic of a professional, they are viewed as a horizontal strand. The emphasis is on individual responsibility and accountability to the consumer of health and nursing care.

Ethics and the Legal Process. This is taught consistently in relation to nursing in accord with professional and legal nursing standards.

Trends: Past, Present, and Future. These trends are taught as evolving in relationship to humanity, society, health, and nursing.

Independent and Interdependent Functions. As a horizontal strand, the concept of being independent and interdependent is developed in relation to the practice of nursing. This emphasizes the autonomy of the nursing profession and the need for being accountable and responsible for the practice of nursing and for taking a leadership role within the health care system.

Role Development. This strand focuses on the socialization into expected behavior patterns that are congruent with the nurse/client relationship.

Health Potential Patterns. This strand focuses on the dynamic patterns of human functioning which help to minimize vulnerability.

Health Promotion, and Maintenance. These are viewed as representing the major activities of the professional practitioner in relation to the client's state of health.

At this point, the theoretical framework is rather dictatorial in its impact. Answer the following questions as you review the placement of the content elements. Note that the clinical nursing courses are given during the third and fourth years and each year has three courses as identified.

1. Will the content elements related to the care of clients who have maximum health be emphasized during the first clinical nursing course?

2. Will the learner utilize the nursing process to initiate change within the health care system during the fifth and sixth nursing courses?

3. Will the emphasis on community assessment as one aspect of the nursing process be during the fourth year?

4. Is the learner initially providing care to the client who has an impaired health state during the second nursing course?

The answer to these questions is yes. If a framework is to assist in the development of level objectives, clarity is essential. Otherwise, there will be confusion, duplication, and vacuums in the content elements. This should become increasingly clear as we later review the developed level objectives. We can view the "whole" of the curriculum rather than focus on the parts and hope that relationships exist.

Table 6.3 shows the relationships among the components of the directive stage of the curriculum process within the context of a developed curriculum. Note that the criteria for evaluating the consistency of the developed curriculum are well supported, the content elements can be seen within the propositions and characteristics, the terms utilized among the components are consistent, and there are no contradictions.

A review of the terminology used supports the need for a glossary of terms to give clarity to their meaning. It is essential that terms such as health, leadership, and human environment be used in a similar manner throughout the program. The

Table 6.3

Relationship of Components Within the Directive Stage

CHARACTERISTICS OF THE GRADUATE	PROPOSITIONS WITHIN THE PHILOSOPHY	THEORETICAL FRAMEWORK		LEVEL OF ACHIEVEMENT
		Content	Process	
Assess and diagnose the health status of individuals, families, groups, and communities; plan implement, and evaluate nursing care in any setting within and outside the health care delivery system.	"Individual's interaction with the health care system. . . ." "Society . . . composed of individuals, families, groups, and communities." "The nursing process. . . ." "Health is. . . ."	Health status of individuals, families, groups, and communities Health care system	Nursing, health promotion, health potential patterns	Application Evaluation
Synthesize theories and/or concepts related to the arts, sciences, and nursing into practice as a professional nurse.	"The practice of professional nursing . . . requires a knowledge base in nursing. The integration of scientific, humanistic, and nursing concepts and theories . . . give direction to this practice."	All theories and concepts	Nursing	Application Synthesis
Provide professional nursing care based on an understanding of the uniquely evolving patterns of human existence in relation to the client's health status and potential.	"Human existence involves behavioral patterns. Health is influenced by inherent capabilities . . . human existence . . . interaction with unique life experience. . . ."	Health status related to human patterns of functioning	Nursing, health promotion, health potential patterns.	Application Analysis

Incorporate the interpersonal process in providing care, nurturance, and protection to individuals, families, groups, and communities in relation to their state of health.	"Nursing is interpersonal and caring...." "Society... composed of individuals, families, groups, and communities." "Health is...."	Interpersonal, health status	Nursing	Comprehension Application
Function as the nucleus of the health care professionals utilizing leadership and interactive concepts and theories to coordinate and collaborate on matters related to nursing care.	"The professional nurse... viewed as nucleus of the health care system... through leadership and interaction skills... with other health and nursing practitioners...."	Leadership Interactive Decision making	Interdependent—independent function, Role	Comprehension
Accept a personal philosophy of professional nursing that incorporates professional responsibility and accountability to, and advocacy for, the consumer of nursing care.	"The emerging role... accountability to the consumer. The professional nurse... as well as an advocate for the consumer."	Nursing	Accountability and responsibility; Ethic and legal process	Organization Conceptualization of a value
Recognize the impact of environmental forces on the health care system.	"Human existence... interact with biological, psychological, social, spiritual, and other forces in the environment." These dynamic forces... placed upon the health care system."	Environmental Political systems		Comprehension
Utilize the change process to	"Human existence... con-	Change	Nursing trends—	Analysis

Table 6.3

Relationship of Components Within the Directive Stage (*continued*)

CHARACTERISTICS OF THE GRADUATE	PROPOSITIONS WITHIN THE PHILOSOPHY	THEORETICAL FRAMEWORK	*LEVEL OF ACHIEVEMENT
influence the environmental forces toward improving health and nursing care as it relates to the emerging role of the professional nurse.	stant change . . . Change in the environment. The emerging role of the nurse. . . ."	past, present and future	Application
Demonstrates responsibility for self-direction in the life-long process of learning by participating in activities that contribute to personal and professional growth.	"The learner has responsibility for independence, self-direction, and reaching a level of self-realization."	Learning	Valuing—preference for a value
		Accountability	
Utilize nursing research to improve practice and gather reliable and accurate data to extend nursing science.	"The practice of professional nursing . . . requires knowledge . . . attainable through research, gives direction to practice."	Nursing Research	Application Evaluation
		Nursing process Research process	

---

*Utilization of Bloom's taxonomy—cognitive and affective domain.

following glossary of terms lists those terms which the faculty feels must be clearly defined in order to implement the curriculum.

Glossary of Terms

CONCEPT	TERMS	DEFINITIONS
Humanity	Human existence	Totality of human experience from conception to physiological death
	Interaction	Mutual or reciprocal action or influence
	Patterns	A composite sample of traits or behaviors which are characterized by rhythm, rate, intensity, duration, and amount
	Spiritual	An internal essence or quality that gives meaning to an individual's life
	Unique	The way individuals differ from each other by virtue of heredity, environment, particular experiences, perception of such experiences, and the manner in which they react to such experiences.
Society	Community	A specific population living within a defined perimeter or a group which has common values, interests, or needs
	Health care system	The organized distribution of services and personnel to meet the health needs of others
	Responsibility	Obligation to fulfill the terms of implied or explicit contractual agreement in accord with professional and legal nursing standards

Glossary of Terms (*continued*)

CONCEPT	TERMS	DEFINITIONS
Health	Depleted health	Alteration in the dynamic pattern of functioning whereby there is the inability to interact with internal and external forces as the result of a temporary or permanent loss of necessary resources
	Health	Dynamic pattern of functioning whereby there is a continued interaction with internal and external forces which result in the optimal use of necessary resources that serve to minimize vulnerabilities
	Health maintenance	The act of protecting and preserving patterns of maximum potential for health
	Health promotion	The advancement of patterns of functioning which foster and/or encourage health
	Impaired health	Alteration in the dynamic pattern of functioning whereby there is a diminished ability to interact with internal and external forces as the result of a reduction in necessary resources
	Maximum potential for health	Ability to achieve or develop the highest pattern of functioning possible within the client's health parameter
	Resource	External or internal source of strength or assistance
	Vulnerability	State of being at risk or susceptible

CONCEPT	TERMS	DEFINITIONS
Nursing	Account-ability	Liability for the extent to which actions taken were consistent with the responsibility for which he/she contracted; it implies that the actual performance will be judged against professionally established codes and standards
	Advocate	One who acts in the interest of the health care consumer
	Caring	To be concerned about or interested in another
	Client	Individual, family, group, or community
	Concept	A complex mental formulation of objects, events, or ideas which can be symbolized by a word label
	Collaboration	A joint effort for the purpose of creating change toward a mutually desired goal
	Coordination	Regulation and combination of effort for harmonious performance
	Consortium	An association with others, which fosters an interdependent relationship, for the achievement of mutual goals
	Human environment	The total of circumstances surrounding an organism; includes living organisms, natural resources, inanimate objects, cosmic elements, and aesthetic factors
	Independent	Not relying on or requiring the support of others for the authority to perform nursing activities

CONCEPT	TERMS	DEFINITIONS
	Leader	A person with foresight who is able to influence others in a positive direction, who is accountable for her or his own beliefs, who is willing and able to take risks, who accepts the concept of power and uses it judiciously
	Leadership	A complex relationship between individuals whereby interpersonal influence is exercised through the process of communication toward the achievement of specific goals
	Nucleus	The central professional in the health care system
	Nurse practitioner	One who practices professional nursing
	Nursing process	A deliberate intellectual activity whereby the practice of nursing is approached in an orderly, systematic manner; it includes the following components:
		Assessment—the process of data collection and analysis which results in a conclusion or nursing diagnosis
		Nursing diagnosis—a statement describing the client's current or potential health status which is based on nursing assessment and projects nursing intervention
		Plan—the determination of what can be done to assist the client; involves mutual goal setting,

CONCEPT	TERMS	DEFINITIONS
		judging priorities, and designing methods to resolve problems and/or promote or maintain health Implementation—action of carrying out the plan Evaluation—appraisal of the client's behavioral changes and goal achievement
	Research	A systematic inquiry to discover facts or test theories in order to obtain valid answers to questions or solutions for problems
	Role	A dyadic relationship which is an actual or expected behavior pattern determined by socialization, including the interaction and interpretation of given norms, status, or position
	Science	An integrated pattern of knowing which includes law, theory, application, and instrumentation in the context of empirical reality
Learning	Educator	A person who is committed to scholarship and research, who is skilled in teaching, who understands and respects the learner, who guides and supports learning

Consistency of meaning *between each of the terms* is important if the definitions are to be useful. Since health is viewed in the context of dynamic patterns, the definitions of depleted and impaired health as well as the definitions of maximum potential for health all relate to the concept of patterns. The glossary of terms is developed in relation to each key concept to facilitate the development and recognition of such relationships.

The course descriptions in Table 6.4 are consistent with the components of the directive stage in their concepts and terminology. The prerequisites also support the theoretical framework and its vertical strands. For example, the majority of science courses are prerequisites to Nursing 211. This supports the propositions within the philosophy that nursing requires a scientific base of knowledge, and it supports the framework which identifies the sciences as prerequisite to the third and fourth years of the program. The descriptions also reflect the content elements within the level and course objectives.

The curriculum requirements in Table 6.5 reflect the combination of the building and progressive models since a minimal amount of the total nursing credits is required during the first two years of the program. A diagram of this is given in Fig. 6.2.

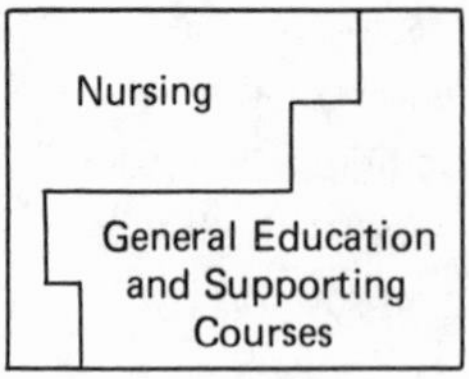

Year		Total Number of Quarter Credits	Percent of Nursing Requirements Per Year	Percent of Nonnursing Requirement
4	Nursing	49	68	32
3		49	61	39
2	General Education and Supporting	46	12	88
1	Courses	50	16	84

Figure 6.2
Summary of Curriculum Requirements

Table 6.4
Course Descriptions

YEAR	COURSE	CREDITS	PREREQUISITES
I	NUR 111 The Health Care System: Its Impact on Professional Nursing - An introductory course oriented toward the role and function of the professional nurse within the health care system.	3	
	NUR 114 Nursing Elective - Special Topics	2 or 3	
II	NUR 211 Scientific and Nursing Concepts and Theories - Concepts and theories from the arts, sciences, and nursing are discussed in terms of their significance to the practice of professional nursing. Included is the comparison of various theories, as well as an orientation to the program's philosophy and theoretical framework.	4	NUR 111, English, General Psychology, Introductory Sociology, Chemistry, Biology, Anatomy, Physiology, Nutrition, Microbiology

Table 6.4

Course Descriptions (*continued*)

YEAR	COURSE		CREDITS	PREREQUISITES
III	NUR 311	(Noted as I, II, and III on Theoretical Framework) Nursing Process: Human Existence and Health I, II, III - Clinical Nursing courses focus on the	9 each quarter	NUR 211, Human Development, Communications, Anthropology
	312	nursing process and individual's, family's ability to interact with environmental forces in relation		NUR 311, Pharmacology, Sociology of Family, Pathophysiology, Abnormal Psychology
	313	to their maximum potential for health. Learning experiences include a variety of settings within and outside the health care system.		NUR 312, NUR 304, Religion, Philosophy
	NUR 304	Foundations of Nursing Research - This course is designed to introduce the junior-level nursing major to the basic elements of the research process, including aspects of statistics. Emphasis	3	NUR 211, NUR 311

will be placed on the relation of research findings to professional nursing practice and the nursing process.

IV	NUR 411	(Noted as IV, V, VI on Theoretical Framework) Nursing Process: Human Existence and Health I, II, III - Clinical Nursing courses oriented	10 each quarter	NUR 313, Political Science
	412	toward the practice of professional nursing with individuals, families, and communities.		NUR 411
	413	Learning experiences emphasize independent and interdisciplinary activities in a variety of environments.		NUR 412
	NUR 414	Nursing Elective - Special Topics	3	Concurrent with NUR 411, 412, or 413
	NUR 415	Independent Study	3	Concurrent with NUR 411, 412, 413

Table 6.5
Requirements in Quarter Credits

YEAR	HUMANITIES ELECTIVES CREDITS	SCIENCE CREDITS	NURSING CREDITS	TOTAL CREDITS
1	English: 8 Communications: 3 Electives: 3	Biology: 4 Chemistry: 9 Psychology: 6 Sociology: 6 Anatomy: 8	Nursing 111: 3	50
2	Electives: 9 Philosophy: 3 Humanities: 3	Nutrition: 3 Physiology: 10 Anthropology: 3 Microbiology: 5	Nursing 211: 4	

	Developmental Psychology: 3 Pharmacology: 3			46
3	Religion: 3 Political Science: 4	Sociology/family: 3 Pathophysiology: 4 Abnormal Psychology: 4	Nursing 311, 312, and 313: 27 Nursing 304: 3	49
4	Electives: 6 Humanities: 6 Philosophy or Religion: 3	-0-	Nursing 411, 412, and 413: 30 Nursing Elective 3	49
TOTAL CREDITS	51	71	71	193

The model is basically consistent with the components of the directive stage which fosters the integration of scientific, humanistic, and nursing concepts and theories as giving direction to nursing practice. Thus, the clinical nursing component is offered during the last two years. The first nursing course which relates to an orientation to professional nursing is not built on scientific knowledge; therefore, it has no prerequisites.

The curriculum design consists of 37 percent nursing and science requirements and 26 percent electives and humanities. Since it is probable that the 18 credits in free electives will also include some science courses, the curriculum may not be adequately balanced and should require more courses in the humanities. Variables which most strongly affect such a design are the prerequisites for the sciences and the general education components required for the degree. For example, pathophysiology requires anatomy and physiology as prerequisites, and chemistry is a prerequisite for nutrition. Also, the general education requirements mandate that three related sciences be taken in sequence.

The specific requirements have evolved from the theoretical framework. Courses in political science, family sociology, and anthropology give credence to the propositions within the concept of society. Similarly, the strong science requirements support the concepts of humanity and health. These requirements also support the notion that nursing as a discipline should be taught by nurse educators and the sciences by the appropriate science faculty. This is demonstrated by requiring nutrition, pharmacology, abnormal psychology, and especially pathophysiology as prerequisite courses to nursing courses rather than teaching such knowledge within the nursing courses.

The level and course objectives reflect the theoretical framework and the characteristics of the graduate. In reviewing these, it should be noted that all curriculum strands are identified and that each nursing course has an objective which was developed from the level objective which was developed from the characteristic. Carefully review the first characteristic and the developed objectives (see also Table 6.6). The following can be noted:

The humanity and society strand is separated so that individuals and families are the focus at the third level and the individual family and community are the focus at the fourth level. The previous components of the strand

Table 6.6

Characteristics of the Graduate in Relation to Level and Course Objectives with Major Strands that Affect Their Development

CHARACTERISTIC	LEVEL 100	LEVEL 200	LEVEL 300	LEVEL 400
Assess and diagnose the health status of individuals, families, and communities. Plan, implement, and evaluate nursing care in any setting within and outside the health care delivery system.	Understanding the present and emerging health care delivery system.	Utilize intellectual processes of critical thinking. Define the components of the nursing process.	Utilize the nursing process to promote maximum potential of individuals and families with maximum and impaired health throughout the life cycle in selected settings within and without the health care delivery system. Utilize the nursing process to promote maximum potential of individuals with depleted health throughout the life cycle in selected settings within the health care delivery system.	Utilize the nursing process to promote maximum potential of individuals, families, and communities having maximum, impaired, or depleted health in selected settings within and without the health care system.

Within the nested structure of LEVEL 300 and LEVEL 400 columns:

LEVEL 300

Course 311
Utilize the nursing process to promote maximum potential of individuals with maximum health throughout the life cycle.

Course 312
Utilize the nursing process to promote maximum potential of families with maximum health throughout the life cycle.
Utilize the nursing process to promote maximum potential of individuals with impaired health throughout the life cycle.

Course 313
Utilize the nursing process to promote maximum potential of individuals with depleted health throughout the life cycle.
Utilize the nursing process to promote maximum potential of impaired families throughout the life cycle.

LEVEL 400

Course 411
Utilize the nursing process to promote maximum potential of families with impaired health.
Utilize the nursing process to promote maximum potential of communities with maximum health.
Utilize the nursing process to promote maximum potential of individuals with multiple health states.

Course 412
Utilize the nursing process to promote maximum potential of communities with impaired health.
Utilize nursing process to promote maximum potential of individuals and families with multiple health states.

Course 413
Utilize the nursing process to promote maximum potential of individuals, families, and communities with multiple health states in selected settings within and without the health care delivery system.

Left-hand strand labels (vertical):

Course 413, 412, 411, 313, 312, 311

Individual, Family, Humanity and Society, Community

Maximum, Impaired, Depleted, Multiple Health States

Promotion, Maintenance, Health

Nursing Process — Health Potential Patterns (appears twice)

are repeated during the fourth level since the state of health changes. This is essential to ensure that the family which has the status of impaired or depleted health is within the objectives at the fourth level. Thus, matching the *humanity and society* strands with the *health states* strand assists in the development of the objectives. The sequence at the 300 level is: individual with maximum health, families with maximum health, individuals with impaired health, individuals with depleted health, families with impaired health. The same approach is used at the 400 level.

The horizontal strand—the nursing process—is consistently used to direct all objectives. Thus, the nursing process supports the vertical strands which direct the content elements.   /

The objectives closely relate to the propositions within the philosophy.

The objectives have a strong impact on curriculum requirements. For example, pathophysiology, family sociology, and abnormal psychology need to be parallel or prerequisite courses to Nursing 312 since the objectives focus on the impaired individuals and the healthy family.

The first level relates to understanding within the cognitive domain; all other objectives require application and evaluation since the nursing process includes both these components.

In reviewing the content map it can be observed that the content elements are consistent with the components of the directive and formative stages. The map differentiates the content elements from one course to the other (see Table 6.7).

Thus, the nursing curriculum is developed within a theoretical framework that is formed and supported by vertical and horizontal strands which support the philosophy, purposes, and objectives of the program. The concepts reflected in the strands are used with the characteristics of the graduate as

Table 6.7
Content Map (Content Elements)

	NUR 311	NUR 312	NUR 313	NUR 411	NUR 412	NUR 413
Focus	Individual w/maximum health throughout the life span; Nursing process. Coordinating role of the nurse	Individual w/impaired health; Family w/maximum health	Individual w/impaired health; Individual w/depleted health; Families w/short-term impaired health	Families w/impaired health; Communities w/maximum health; Collaborating role of the nurse	Family w/depleted health; Communities w/impaired health	Family w/depleted health; Community w/depleted health; Comprehensive health care
Concepts and Patterns	Wellness and health; Developmental; Accountability and responsibility; Values; Nutrition; Interpersonal; Peplau; Orem; Holism; Humanistic; Coordination; Assertiveness; Communication; Learning; Wiedenbach; Orlando; Rogers	Self-concept; Immobility; Group dynamics; Communication w/groups; Behavior modification; Levine; Body image Deprivation; Family theory system; Orem; King; Stress	Need; Pain; Research; Henderson; Orlando; Death and dying; Epidemiology; Euthanasia; Loss; Crisis; Hall; Abdellah; Nightingale	Collaboration; Community; Organizational; Role; Crisis; Interpersonal; Roy	World health; Leadership; Ecology; Economics; Epidemiology; Poverty	Disaster; Change; Decision making; Political; Systems; Evaluation; Suicide

Table 6.7
Content Map (Content Elements) (continued)

	NUR 311 (continued)	NUR 312 (continued)	NUR 313 (continued)	NUR 411 (continued)	NUR 412 (continued)	NUR 413 (continued)
M a j o r	Nursing process w/ healthy individual	Nursing process w/ healthy family	Nursing process w/ individual w/depleted health potential	Nursing process w/ community w/ maximum health potential	Nursing process w/ community w/ impaired health	Nursing process w/ community w/ depleted health
	Assessment-data collection, interview	Normal family relationships	Nursing process w/ individual w/ short-term, self-limiting problems	Nursing process w/ family w/impaired health	World health problems, Epidemics, endemics, ecology populations	Quality assurance
	Analysis	Preparing for parenthood		Battered family		Disasters
	Diagnosis	Parenting	Nursing process w/ impaired family and nontraditional relationships	Substance abuse	Nursing process w/ family w/depleted health	Triage
	Plan-goal and intervention	Family food patterns		Exceptional children	Infertility	Alternate health care systems
C o n t e n t	Evaluation	Family planning (contraception)	Threats to life	Health care delivery system	Adoption	
	Health promotion and protection	Nursing process w/ individuals w/ long-term rehabilitation	Death and dying	Peer review	Emergencies	
	Teaching		Inability to cope	Conflict	Human sexuality	
	Immunization		Apathy, depression, paranoia, powerlessness, hopelessness,			
	Coping w/normal fear, anxiety, stress	coping w/fear, anxiety, stress, dependency, psychosomatic, anger, frustration, confusion, scapegoating	Genetic counseling			
A r e a s	Self-evaluation					
	Nutrition of healthy individual					

Learning Experiences

Tapes for interviewing, communication, assessment
Health history, screening skills
Lab experience for assessment skills (hands on)
Nursing process with healthy individual in structured settings

Pick up individual client
Nursing process w/ healthy family in structured setting
Group experiences
Teaching plans individuals groups
Family teaching
Nutrition programs
Nursing process w/individual w/impaired health

Nutrition and stress
Pre and post-op nutrition,
Infant feeding
Continue w/ healthy family
Outpatient experiences
Crisis centers
Short-term surgery
Lab experiences with technical skills

Community process   Impaired Community   Triage, disaster activities
Health department activities
Community experiences include: group project, agencies, professionals, board meetings, hospice, clinics
Impaired family caseload
Seminar
Structured settings (individual family)
Mental health: outpatient, inpatient, group, organizations
Children (all ages): well, sick (short-term, chronic, critical), death
Childbearing: prenatal, birthing, postnatal, newborn, clinics
Adults: well, short-term, chronic, crisis
Supportive lab experiences, as needed

guidelines to develop specific behavioral undergraduate level objectives which in turn guide and direct learning goals in the curriculum. The level objectives are then used to develop course objectives which guide the selection of learning experiences. This progression of curriculum development from design to implementation assures that the philosophy, purposes, and objectives of the program function within the theoretical framework.

Next we need to look at the learner and the learning process. The key points here are the learner, the educator, the knowledge, and the environment (see Fig. 6.3). The interaction of these four points has a profound effect on whether or not the curriculum that has been developed will achieve its goal of assisting the learner to meet the characteristics of the graduate. Implied in that knowledge, which could be identified as the content elements, is the central focus of both the faculty and the learner, and the environment surrounds the other three concepts. The environment should be viewed in a limited sense in relation to a classroom and in a broader sense in relation to the total educational institution, the community at large, and even the universe. It is possible to place the center of attention on the learner by placing the learner between knowledge and the faculty. This would, in a sense, support the belief that the faculty and the knowledge should

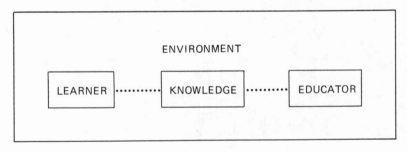

Figure 6.3
Interaction Among Learner, Educator, Knowledge, and the Environment

be directed to the learner. The difference is a significant one in terms of the role of faculty and learner. If the responsibility for learning is the student's, and if the faculty provides a format through a well-developed curriculum plan for the knowledge to be achieved, then the concept of knowledge is central. Also, this framework acknowledges that both faculty and students use and develop knowledge as a basis for the practice of the discipline or the education of the learner.

Whether a curriculum is successful or not depends on two things. One is the *characteristics* of each point which support or hinder the implementation of the developed curriculum and the other is the match and/or *interrelativeness* among the four points: learner, knowledge, educator, and environment. When problems occur in terms of the ability of the learner to achieve the characteristics and objectives, a careful analysis utilizing the conceptual model previously mentioned will give strong clues to their causes. Assume that a curriculum has been developed by a faculty and its implementation is to begin within a few months. What characteristics of each point would be *most* supportive or nonsupportive of such a curriculum endeavor?

Knowledge

The characteristics of knowledge relate to the content elements in the form of concepts/theories, skills, and attitudes that have been identified as significant to the discipline. Such knowledge needs to be easily *available* in some form such as in books, journals, or films so that it can be taught and be useful to the learner. For example, textbooks would need to focus on nursing as a process discipline and human existence in forms of behavioral patterns. Nursing research, which adds to the body of knowledge of the discipline, must provide the faculty and learner which updated nursing theories and concepts. The process orientation which focuses on health promotion rather than on illness would require that we have the knowledge essential to educate for practice within that framework. There must be a difference between how one educates for the acquisition of specific concepts/theories and how one educates for the acquisition of a skill. The processes taught must be useful in all nursing situations. The following questions might assist the faculty in assessing the status of the knowledge it needs in order to educate.

1. Can the knowledge be found and is it easily available?

2. Is such knowledge well-developed and/or researched so that it is functional for educational purposes?

3. Is the knowledge within the framework of nursing as a discipline and as reflected within the curriculum?

The answers to these questions should generally be positive for real success. If there is concern, ways have to be identified to allow for any weaknesses in the educational process. For example, since nursing frameworks/theories are seldom well researched and documented in terms that will facilitate the educational process, they need to be presented in that context to the learner. Thus, it is essential that the student be exposed to multiple frameworks to ensure a breadth of knowledge rather than a depth within a loosely developed framework. Also, if a specific text does not relate to the knowledge, several texts may have to be used to teach broad concepts/theories as dictated by the curriculum. In other words, medical model textbooks would be totally inappropriate in the context of a nursing model curriculum. The knowledge would not be congruent.

The Educator

The characteristics of the educator are the most crucial in terms of their impact on the implementation of the curriculum. Most frequently, their characteristics are the major force as to whether there will be success or failure. The knowledge the educator brings to educational endeavors is the key factor that will influence the selection of the content elements during the development of the curriculum and it is also the key factor in what the learner will be taught. Educators who as a group and individually are secure because they either have the knowledge or are willing to learn the knowledge that has been identified within these content elements will be successful even if the other three concepts within this framework are only fairly supportive. Other characteristics relate to their ability to use effective group and interpersonal processes. An open communication system among the faculty and planned time to share concerns and problems are essential. The educators' perception of their role in the implementation plan needs to be discussed so that its impact on them as individuals will be more fully realized. Commitment to the decisions made during the curriculum development stages needs to be verbalized frequently. Again, there are important questions to ask, for example:

1. Is the educator adequately knowledgeable about the content elements?

2. Will faculty members be supportive of continuing education if it is essential for their development?

3. Are the educators cognizant and realistic about the impact the curriculum will have on them as a group and as individuals?

4. Does the educator's practice and educational background support the curriculum model developed?

5. Does the educator give top priority to the effective implementation of the curriculum?

6. Within the context of the developed nursing model, will the educator prepared as a medical model specialist (such as medical-surgical or psychiatric nursing) be willing and able to resist holding onto territories of medical knowledge such as pathophysiology and focus on teaching nursing?

Again, the more positive the responses to these questions, the greater the degree of success. Basic are a sense of involvement and commitment and a willingness to learn. The last question is one of the most critical and demands honest and open interactions in regard to any curriculum which moves away from the medical model approach.

The Learner

The learners' characteristics relate to their ability to be successful in achieving the developed course objectives. The characteristics involve their intellectual capacity, their ability to modify or develop certain attitudes, and their ability to perform psychomotor skills. For example, if the curriculum focuses on theoretical and abstract knowledge and requires synthesis, the learner must have the ability to think or learn to think at a higher level than just acquiring facts. Also, involved is the learner's ability to be acculturated into the discipline of nursing as developed within the philosophy. There needs to be congruence between the learner's beliefs and/or philosophy of nursing and learning and that which is supported within the curriculum. The assessment of the learner can take various forms, for example, prediagnostic tools related to intellectual ability, but generally we need to recognize that we are without adequate tools. We usually function with hindsight rather than foresight in terms of problems that may arise. This provides us with the data to make changes and is done in the context of both formative and summative evaluations. Within that context the following questions can be asked:

1. Is the learner able to articulate a philosophy of nursing that is supportive of the curriculum?

2. Is the learner's own self-assessment of her or his ability to achieve similar to the faculty's and adequate for the achievement of the objectives?

We need to do much more research in nursing education if we are to better assess learners in terms of their ability to practice within a nursing framework. Until we do this, the best we can do is ask such questions.

The Environment

As noted within the conceptual model, the characteristics within the environment have a direct impact on the knowledge, learner, and educator. Within the learner's immediate environment there have to be adequate facilities, equipment, and faculty to implement the curriculum. Within the institution there has to be support for the curriculum model that has been developed. Within the community there have to be adequate clinical facilities that will facilitate the learning of the behaviors supported by the curriculum and its objectives. Also, nurse leaders within the community must be supportive or at least cognizant and accepting of the implications of the curriculum in the practice of nursing within that community. Another environmental factor involves the standards set by state and national organizations, for example, state boards and the National League for Nursing. The curriculum needs to support the trends in nursing and nursing education. Thus, the characteristics within any of these environments can be viewed from a philosophical or resource framework. Within the philosophical context, the standards in terms of quality control play an important role. For example, the qualifications of the faculty and the criteria for rank, promotion, and tenure all have a strong impact. Resources are often viewed in terms of economics and clinical facilities and need to be specifically assessed within the context of the specific curriculum. Again, the following questions should be asked:

1. Are the resources within the environment appropriate and adequate in terms of quality and quantity to implement the curriculum?

2. Is there significant philosophical support within and outside the immediate environment to facilitate learning in the context of the curriculum?

Actually, it would be unusual if an outright "yes" were given in answer to each of these questions. A search for the degree of positiveness may have greater validity. The identification of the resources available and an assessment of the philosophical support need to be examined carefully and viewed from a positive and negative framework to understand their environmental impact on the curriculum.

The assessment of the relationships and a total view of the interplay between each of these points are essential since neither functions in isolation. Strengths or weaknesses in the characteristics of any one point will have a significant effect on the others. For example, without adequate available knowledge in a useful form, difficulties will arise for both students and faculty. Inadequately prepared faculty or learners who are not sufficiently acculturated into the system will tend to create a stressful environment. Thus, interrelativeness should be analyzed before any decisions are made on changes or on the use of resources so that priorities can be established to strengthen the potential for success. Professional judgments on the part of the educators with input from the learner and from the community within and outside the immediate environment are essential in an environment in which open communication methods are encouraged. Questions for discussion might reflect the following:

1. Is the environment perceived conducive to the acquisition of knowledge by the educator and learner?

2. Does the learner support the educator's perception of the knowledge that has been selected as foundational to practicing nursing within the community?

3. Does the educator's perception of the characteristics of the learner enhance the acquisition of knowledge within the environment?

4. Is there a positive relationship between the major focuses identified within the knowledge area (content elements) and the educator's, learner's, and the community's perceived values in terms of these priorities?

Since perceptions and values are difficult to assess, the above questions should be viewed as a basis for further and continued analysis. As the curriculum is implemented, there should be frequent discussions in order to "get a handle" on these points. All too often there is little or no communication in some structured environments and hence there is a lack of clarity and understanding. In the nonstructured environment there is often a rumor mode of communication which heightens the stress created by change and at any given point causes a real contamination of the developed curriculum.

Summary

A sample curriculum is offered in order to facilitate understanding of the curriculum process. It is also used to assess the consistency between and among stages of the developed curriculum.

7

The Registered
or Practical Nurse
as a Transfer Student
into a Degree Program

In dealing with transfer students, it is essential that the faculty accepts the following assumptions as general guidelines for action. These will be discussed in more detail throughout the chapter.

1. The *curriculum process* must be utilized to better meet the individual needs of transfer students.

2. Transfer students *differ substantially* in their characteristics; thus generalizations are difficult to make.

3. Transfer students require a *greater degree of assessment,* especially during the initial phases of their program.

4. Transfer students must *meet the same requirements* for the degree as other students.

5. The more individualized the program, the *greater the investment* of time and other resources of the faculty.

Planning Prior to the Development
of the Curriculum

Decisions that must be made prior to the development of the curriculum relate to the types of students that will be admitted to the program. Such decisions must be based on the educational institution's goals and the community needs that have been identified. An institution committed to the admission of current high school graduates only and oriented to preparing graduates majoring in the humanities differs substantially from a community-oriented institution that wants to meet the needs of all potential students within that area. Decisions must be based on the answers to the following questions:

1. What types of transfer students are the potential candidates for admission?

2. What are the particular educational needs of these transfer students and are resources for meeting these needs available within the institution?

3. What are the economic implications as related to the acceptance or nonacceptance of certain transfer students?

4. Are there adequate numbers of potential students to project a viable enrollment over the next five or ten years?

5. Are there adequate clinical and other facilities to handle these transfer students?

6. What other institutions in the area already meet the needs of these transfer students?

7. If various types of transfer students are to be admitted, should a ratio of the different types be developed?

There are many choices from which an institution can decide what types of students are to be accepted. Such decisions must be strongly influenced by the particular institution's characteristics. The following table shows examples of the relationship between institutional characteristics and the type of student admitted:

Once the institution has decided which type(s) of students to admit, the faculty can then begin to develop the curriculum with a clear idea of the type of student population it will serve. This should help to ensure that each of the curriculum components is supportive of the goals of the program.

TYPE OF STUDENT ADMITTED	INSTITUTIONAL CHARACTERISTICS
Admit only students directly from high school	Strong commitment to meeting the needs of high school graduates with an emphasis on humanistic and/or career development
Admit only associate degree graduates	Strong commitment to the building of one career goal on another across the entire institution Within a community that has many community colleges offering associate degrees, there is usually a close articulation between institutions
Admit only diploma graduates to baccalaureate program *or* practical nurse graduates into baccalaureate or associate degree program	Strong commitment to and acceptance of the concept of lifelong learning and other forms of continuing education for the mature learner Flexibility in offering examinations for credit and providing opportunities for all students to take national tests for credit

TYPE OF STUDENT ADMITTED	INSTITUTIONAL CHARACTERISTICS
	for the general education requirements Resources must be available to develop evaluation tools specifically oriented to measure incoming students for placement within and outside the curriculum requirements
Admit nongraduated generic students from other degree programs	Flexible course requirements, especially in the sciences and nursing
Admit any combination of the above types of transfer students and high school graduates	A large institution which has a wide range of programs that offers credit-by-examination and is committed to all types of student

Curriculum Development and the Transfer Student

Since the *philosophy* of the program has a profound effect on all the components of the curriculum, it must reflect a clear commitment through its developed propositions as to the type of student that will be admitted to the program. For example, philosophical statements that emphasize the building of the professional nursing knowledge on content elements (knowledge, skills, and attitudes) focusing on individuals, illness, and the technology of nursing would be more supportive of the acceptance of associate degree and diploma graduates, since this is the usual framework of their previous educational preparation. Conversely, philosophical statements that speak to the need for a strong humanistic and scientific *base* of knowledge *prior* to the learning of the nursing content tend to be less supportive of developing curricula for certain types of transfer students. When such graduates attempt to articulate into programs designed to provide scientific knowledge prior to the learning of nursing content, difficulty arises in requiring transfer students to take several science courses prior to beginning the nursing sequence. However individual assessment of a student's academic background can minimize many of these difficulties.

Note the following propositions in terms of their support or relative nonsupport for the nurse transfer student:

> Professional nursing is a composite of technical and theoretical knowledge, skills, and attitudes which enhance the provision of quality nursing care.

> Professional nursing is a human interaction based on the strong scientific and theoretical knowledge required to provide quality nursing care.

The first proposition is much more supportive of upper division registered nurse programs while the second proposition is more supportive of the generic programs. Thus, each proposition should be carefully analyzed by an objective educator to ensure that it gives support to the types of students who will enter and progress through the program.

The *theoretical framework*, with its horizontal and vertical strands, can be instrumental in facilitating the faculty's development of the content elements that are essential for the transfer students. It provides a visual picture of the level at which the student should enter the program and the relationship between the previous educational program and the point of entry into the baccalaureate program. In other words, as the student's knowledge, skills, and attitudes are being assessed, the faculty can see how they fit into the program by examining the theoretical framework.

The theoretical framework is particularly helpful to those programs that offer both an associate degree and an articulated baccalaureate degree nursing program. Here the vertical strands become instrumental in differentiating the content elements between the two programs. Figure 7.1 shows an example of the use of a theoretical framework to document the differences between an associate degree program and a baccalaureate degree program. Note the following:

The nursing process, a horizontal strand, remains the same. This is not to assume that the emphasis of each of the components of the nursing process is identical within the two levels. For example, a greater emphasis should be given to implementation on the first and second levels and diagnosis and evaluation on the third and fourth levels.

The vertical strands of health, role, research, and humanity and society provide for a different emphasis between the two degree programs. Admittedly, there may be some overriding emphasis between levels two and three such as the focus on individuals. This is necessary since the first two years do not provide the necessary content elements for the promotion of health of the individual.

This method of setting up a theoretical framework is also helpful to those programs that do not have the first two levels and that only admit registered nurse students at the upper division. The faculty can utilize the content elements identified at levels one and two to develop credit-by-examination for students prior to their placement into the program. This is especially helpful in providing examinations for diploma graduates who do not have transferable credits.

The *characteristics of the graduate* and *level and course objectives* are similarly developed for all types of programs. In institutions that offer both the associate and baccalaureate degrees, the objectives developed at the second level become the characteristics of the associate degree graduate as well

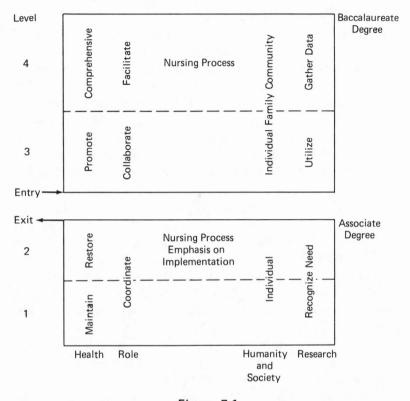

Figure 7.1

Segment of a Theoretical Framework for a Nursing Program Offering Associate and Baccalaureate Degrees

as those characteristics to be validated by the student transferring into the baccalaureate program. Since the characteristics reflect those behaviors that are expected of the graduates of a specific program, nationally developed evaluation tools are generally not reliable unless they in fact do measure the student's ability in relation to the developed characteristics. Since the components of the directive stage of curriculum development differ substantially from program to program, it is highly unlikely that nationally developed tools can be reliable as an assessment tool.

Evaluation tools can be developed specifically to measure the content elements within each objective for either the level or course objectives and ideally for both. It is feasible to develop level examinations for credit that would allow the student to gain credit for multiple nursing courses at one time. As noted in the discussion of curriculum evaluation, such tools are helpful to identify the strengths and weaknesses of the curriculum. Thus, the same evaluative tools can be used for both individual student and curriculum evaluation in certain circumstances.

The *curriculum design* can facilitate the faculty's ability to deal with transfer students. The greater the variety of transfer students admitted to a particular program, the more difficult it will be to create a flexible curriculum design to meet the needs of all students. The sequencing of courses, for example, can create difficulties if the courses are built on multiple prerequisites. The prerequisite requirements can cause the transfer student to have to remain in the program for long periods of time, often on a part-time basis. This does not happen to the high school graduate admitted to the program. Each transfer student's transcript must be individually analyzed to see if the student has met the prerequisite requirement by alternate means.

When totally free electives are a significant portion of the requirements, students with valid transfer credits can receive the greatest amount of transfer benefits for previous college work. For example, some associate degree nursing courses could be utilized to fulfill free elective requirements in a baccalaureate program. Free electives also create a greater degree of flexibility within the program of studies essential to meeting individual needs.

For programs that admit registered nurses exclusively, the parallel curriculum design (see Chapter 3) is most feasible since it provides flexibility and a balanced mixture of nursing, support courses, and general education requirements throughout the program. The parallel curriculum design is helpful in dealing with transfer students since they usually need additional content in all three areas.

The proper development of the components of the *functional stage* of the curriculum process can be most helpful if done with an adequate investment in time and effort. Careful consideration of the needs of the types of students in the program should be reflected in the approaches to content and teaching methods. Instead of making assumptions about students' previous knowledge and experiences, data should be gathered continuously in order to verify the students' abilities in relation to the content being offered. An investment in the development of valid and reliable evaluation tools is essential since these tools reflect the content elements within the course objectives and can be appropriately utilized to give transfer students credit. Thus, credit-by-examination tools are the same as those comprehensive final examinations which are given to all students who take the course for credit. Implied here is that *all* content elements must be evaluated, including clinical skills. Thus, clinical evaluation of the transfer student must be the same as that for all other students in the program.

The curriculum development process can facilitate the program's ability to deal with the student population *if* the educators recognize their responsibility to pattern the program accordingly. It is when the transfer student is either not considered in the development of the program, or considered as an appendage without much recognition, that conflicts and frustration will occur for faculty and students.

Policies Affecting the Transfer Student

Since the development of policies affecting transfer students is strongly influenced by professional standards, legal requirements, and the policies developed by the educational institution, policies cannot be developed in isolation and they cannot differ from other institutional policies that apply to other groups of students. When policies for transfer students are incongruent with those that apply to students admitted from high school, difficulties arise. The development of appropriate policies should be based on educational standards and not on political factors.

The following guidelines should be used to develop policies for transfer students:

1. *Policies need to be clearly written and openly communicated to all faculty and students.* Policies that apply to transfer students should be designed to ensure that they achieve the same educational objectives and learning opportunities as any other group of students. Policies that are not clear tend to confuse both faculty and students and lead to the assumption that transfer students are treated differently, which, of course, creates an unhealthy environment for learning. At times, litigation is threatened or carried out because a student feels that her or his rights have been denied.

2. *Policies need to be modified when appropriate rationale is identified.* Since transfer students differ substantially as individuals, and group characteristics may vary from time to time, constant analysis of the effects of established policies is essential. A lack of policy or the rigid application of policies is equally damaging to the institution as well as to students.

3. *Credit-by-examination policies must differ from those policies that are developed for independent or tutorial study approaches.* Credit-by-examination evaluates the student's knowledge, skills, and attitudes as related to course objectives that have *already* been achieved by the individual. Independent study reflects the ability of the student to learn independently in order to achieve those objectives: tutorial approaches require the faculty to teach on a one-to-one basis to facilitate the learner. Both independent study and the tutorial approach require a different set of guidelines and policies than does the credit-by-examination approach. The resources necessary for each of these approaches are also quite different (tutorial methods are more costly).

4. *All students in the program, whether they are admitted with or without previous education or experience, should have the same opportunities to earn credit-by-examination.* There is a tendency to allow only certain groups of students, such as registered nurses, the opportunity to take credit-by-examination and for nursing credits only. This is an unnecessarily rigid approach since the issue is whether the student can demonstrate

the ability to meet the objectives either by taking examination or by taking the course. The ability to take credit-by-examination should not be based on the student's ability to pass a state board examination, as is the case for the registered nurse student. It should be based on the student's own assessment of her or his knowledge, attitudes, and skills. Thus, any student should be allowed the opportunity to earn credit by whatever methods are available in the institution as long as state board requirements are also met.

5. *The vast majority of the curriculum requirements should be offered for credit-by-examination, particularly those in nursing.* Nursing programs frequently only allow students the opportunity to take credit-by-examination for those courses that the faculty perceives to be similar to the students' previous education and/or experience. This tendency often results in policies that allow for credit-by-examination for the initial few nursing courses. This approach does not adequately allow for individual differences and it inappropriately generalizes about a student population. Science courses should also be offered by credit-by-examination. Evaluation tools that demonstrate accomplishment of objectives in courses other than nursing should be developed by the faculty in the discipline for which the tool is used.

6. *Prior to taking any credit-by-examination, the student must meet all prerequisite requirements for the course.* Since the curriculum is developed to support the concept of progressive learning, it is essential that the student be required to take all prerequisite courses or other required courses prior to taking the examination. This will facilitate the student's ability to pass the tests since it provides the foundation from which the tests were developed. For example, if several science courses are required prior to taking a certain nursing course, the student should not be allowed to take the nursing course examination until the science courses are either challenged by examination or taken for credit.

7. *Policies must be congruent with other related policies within the educational institution.* No policy related to transfer students in nursing should be in contradiction to any policy

within the institution. This is important if the nursing program is to remain an integral and accepted part of the institution, as well as essential in terms of various accreditation organizations such as the North Central or Middle State Accreditation Association. If policies vary, there must be a clear rationale based on appropriate data for the need and purpose for such exceptions. For example, nursing programs cannot offer blanket credit to registered nurse students if all other students in the institution are required to validate knowledge through either institutional evaluation tools or those developed nationally. Unless the institution permits the transfer of credit for lower division course work as equivalent to upper division course work, it is inappropriate for nursing programs to transfer associate degree level nursing courses as equivalent to baccalaureate level nursing courses. Naturally no course should be considered equivalent unless it is equivalent according to faculty judgment.

Summary

The greater the variety of types of students accepted into the nursing program, the more difficult it will be for the faculty to meet the needs of individual students. Conversely, the more limited the type of student admitted, the easier it will be to set up a curriculum to meet an individual student's particular needs. The curriculum components and program policies should be developed with a clear understanding and assessment of the particular student population that will best be served by the educational institution with which the nursing program is affiliated.

Glossary of Terms

Approaches to Content

The model or organizational pattern of content elements which is derived from the directive stage and which gives order to the functional stage of the curriculum process.

Beliefs

Accepted opinions or convictions of truth not necessarily supported by scientific knowledge.

Characteristics of the Graduate

A list of those behaviors, stated as objectives, which reflect the expected knowledge, skills, and attitudes of graduates of a particular program.

Concept

An idea, notion, or abstract mental image derived from an individual's perceptual experience.

Consistency

The extent to which all components of each stage in the curriculum process show relationships between and among each other and support one another in a logical, reasonable way.

Content Elements

Concepts, theories, knowledge, propositions, skills, and attitudes that are identified within the theoretical framework.

Content Map

An outline of the content elements in an appropriate sequence for each nursing course; it also includes the major focus and major concepts, theories, and patterns considered in each course.

Course Outline

The contract between faculty and students specifying faculty and student responsibilities for a particular course. It includes the course description, course objectives, content elements, teaching methods, and evaluation methods for learning and grading.

Course Objectives

Statements of expected behaviors of learners to be demonstrated upon completion of a specific course. The statements are developed from the level objectives.

Credit-by-examination

A method of evaluation for students who feel they have the knowledge, skills, and attitudes gained from other courses or life experiences by which they can demonstrate their competency and gain credit for the course without taking the course. It cannot be used by students who have previously failed the course or by those who have audited the course, and it is not synonymous with independent study or auto-tutorial instruction.

Curriculum Design

The organization and sequencing of course requirements and learning experiences which comprise the total program.

Curriculum Evaluation

A systematic method to validate that the curriculum accomplishes what it was designed for in relation to the characteristics of the graduate. It focuses on the mean achievement scores of students by using aggregate data and it is used by faculty in making decisions about curriculum changes or revisions.

Curriculum Philosophy

A speculative and analytical statement of beliefs about the discipline, including theoretical propositions, which is developed in the directive stage of the curriculum process and serves as the foundation for all other stages and activities of the process.

Curriculum Process

A systematic approach to the development of the learning components of the discipline. It includes four stages: the directive stage, the formative stage, the functional stage, and the evaluation stage.

Directive Stage of the Curriculum Process

The first stage of the curriculum process. It consists of four components: the philosophy, the glossary of terms, the characteristics of the graduate, and the theoretical framework.

Evaluation for Grading

Periodic assessment of the students' achievement of the learning objectives to support progression in the program. It uses formally planned and teacher-developed tools which provide long-range feedback relating to multiple learning experiences.

Evaluation for Learning

Continuous assessment of the students' achievement that enhances the concept of progressive learning and provides immediate feedback relating to a limited learning experience.

Evaluative Stage of the Curriculum Process

The fourth and last stage of the curriculum process. It contains three components: input, throughput, and output.

Formative Stage of the Curriculum Process

The second stage of the curriculum process. It consists of three components: the curriculum design and requirements, the level and course objectives, and the content map.

Functional Stage of the Curriculum Process

The third stage of the curriculum process. It consists of three components: approaches to content, teaching methodology and learning experiences, and validation of learning.

Glossary of Terms

A list of terms and their definitions as developed by a particular faculty. The terms stem from the philosophy and give clarity to the concepts used in the curriculum process.

Horizontal Strands

Process-oriented threads identified in the theoretical framework that are constantly used and reinforced throughout each nursing course in the curriculum.

Input

The initial part of curriculum evaluation. It defines those traits expected of students upon entry into the program and focuses on competencies that support achieving the characteristics of the graduate.

Integrated Nursing-Health Model Approach to Content

An approach that focuses on nursing as a practice discipline with a strong foundation in the nursing theories/concepts which guide practice.

Key Concepts of the Discipline

Concepts that give meaning to and define the nature of the discipline and which are agreed upon by a particular faculty.

Learning Experiences

Activities planned by the faculty with student input to assist students in meeting specific objectives.

Level Objectives

Statements of expected behaviors of the learner to be achieved at specific time intervals in the progression of the program, generally one-year intervals. Level objectives are developed from one or more of the characteristics of the graduate and reflect the theoretical framework.

Medical-Model Approach to Content

An approach that emphasizes medical specialties and a disease/illness orientation. It reflects the belief that medical science applied to the nursing process is integral to the discipline of nursing.

Output

The longitudinal part of curriculum evaluation that examines the traits of graduates of the program in terms of the characteristics of the graduate.

Process

A series of progressive stages in which interdependent activities have a specific purpose. It has the characteristics of being systematic, logical, dynamic, and spiraled.

Proposition

A testable statement showing a relationship between two or more concepts.

Semimedical Model Approach to Content

An approach that emphasizes a common core concept, such as stress/adaptation, which can be used to unify the medical-model specialty concepts. It reflects the belief that unifying the medical specialties leads to a conceptualization of the discipline of nursing.

Teaching Methodology

All teaching activities and learning experiences developed by the faculty with student input to facilitate the students' achievement of the objectives. It includes all classroom, laboratory, and independent learning experiences.

Theoretical Framework

The structuring of the content elements derived from the philosophy in such a way as to ensure systematic implementation of the curriculum philosophy. It contains horizontal (process) and vertical (content) strands which are used as the basis for further development of the curriculum.

Theory

A complex set of relationships between and among concepts. It involves propositions, facts, principles, and laws useful to analyze, predict, describe, explain, and/or control phenomena.

Throughput

The intermediate part of curriculum evaluation that refers to the assessment of all activities related to the cognitive, affective, and psychomotor learning that takes place while the student is in the program.

Transfer Student

A student who has completed course work at one institution and who wishes to receive credit for previously completed work toward a degree in the same or another institution. Specific reference here is to the student who is a licensed practical nurse or who is a registered nurse and is seeking admission into a baccalaureate nursing program.

Vertical Strands

Content threads identified in the theoretical framework which are used to identify and plan progressive learning experiences that build one upon the other throughout all the nursing courses.

Bibliography

Introduction

Bowman, Rosemary, and Culpepper, Rebecca. "Power: Rx for Change," *American Journal of Nursing*, 74: 1053–1056, June, 1974.

Chinn, Peggy L., editor. *"Advances in Nursing Science,"* Nursing Education Issue, 3: April, 1981.

Cosper, Bonnie. "Coping with an Increased Student-Faculty Ratio," *American Journal of Nursing.* 76: 1642–1645, October, 1976.

Culpepper, Rebecca C. "The Nurse's Involvement in Legislation and Public Relations," in *Building for the Future.* Kansas City, American Nurses' Association, 1975.

Driscoll, Veronica. "Liberating Nursing Practice," *Nursing Outlook*, 20: 24–28, January, 1972.

Haase, Patricia. "Pathways to Practice—Part I," *American Journal of Nursing*, 65: 806–809, May, 1965.

———. "Pathways to Practice—Part II," *American Journal of Nursing*, 76: 950–954, June, 1976.

Jacox, Ada. "Address to the Next Generation," *Nursing Outlook*, 26: 38–41, January, 1978.

Kohnke, Mary. "The Nurses Responsibility to the Consumer," *American Journal of Nursing*, 78: 440–442, March, 1978.

McClure, Margaret L. "The Long Road to Accountability," *Nursing Outlook*, 26: 47–50, January, 1978.

Ozimek, Dorothy. *The Future of Nursing Education*. New York, National League for Nursing, Publication 15–1581, 1975.

Stanton, M. "Politics, Power, Risk Taking, and Nursing," in J. Williamson, ed., *Current Perspectives in Nursing Education*. St. Louis: C.V. Mosby Co., 1978.

Chapter 1

Bruner, Jerome. *The Process of Education*. New York: Vantage Books, 1963.

English, Fenwick W., and Kaufman, Roger A. *Needs Assessment: A Focus for Curriculum Development*. Washington, D.C., Association for Supervision and Curriculum Development, 1975, pp. 28–29.

Fischbach, Frances M. "Personal Growth and Learning of Students in an Open-Ended Clinical Experience: A Motivational Philosophy," *Journal of Nursing Education*, 16: 30–33, February, 1977.

Heidie, W.S. "Nursing and Women's Liberation—A Parallel," *American Journal of Nursing*, 73: 824–827, May, 1973.

Malarkey, Louise. "The Older Student–Stress or Success on Campus," *Journal of Nursing Education*, 18: 15–19, February, 1979.

National League for Nursing. *Criteria for the Appraisal of Baccalaureate and Higher Degree Programs in Nursing*. New York: National League for Nursing, Publication 15–1251, 1977.

Parker, J. Cecil, and Rubin, Louis J. *Process as Content: Curriculum Design and the Application of Knowledge*. Chicago: Rand McNally and Company, 1966.

Taba, Hilda. *Curriculum Development: Theory and Practice*. New York: Harcourt Brace and World, Inc., 1962.

Vaillot, Sister Madeleine Clemence. "Nursing Theory, Levels of Nursing, and Curriculum Development," *Nursing Forum*, 20: 234–249, March, 1970.

Wolf-Wilets, Vivian C., and Nugent, L. Catherine. "A Political Analysis of Curriculum Change," *Nursing Outlook*, 27: 207–211, March, 1979.

Chapter 2

Adelotte, Myrtle K. "Clinical Investigation and the Structure of Knowledge," in Miller, M.H., and Flynn, Beverly, eds., *Current Perspectives in Nursing: Social Issues and Trends*. St. Louis: C.V. Mosby Co., 1977.

Bevis, Em Olivia. *Curriculum Building in Nursing: A Process*, 2nd ed. St. Louis: C.V. Mosby Co., 1978.

Chater, Shirley S. "Philosophy versus Framework–A Conceptual Framework for Curriculum Development," *Nursing Outlook*, 23: 428–433, July, 1975.

Conley, Virginia C. *Curriculum and Instruction in Nursing*. Boston: Little, Brown and Co., 1973, pp. 341–388.

Daubenmire, M. Jean, and King, Imogene: "Nursing Process Models: A Systems Approach," *Nursing Outlook*, 21: 512–517, August, 1973.

del Bueno, Dorothy J. "Competency Based Education," *Nurse Educator*, 3: 10–14, May-June, 1978.

Derdiarian, Anayis K. "Education: A Way to Theory Construction in Nursing," *Journal of Nursing Education*, 18: 36–47, February, 1979.

Donaldson, Sue K., and Crowley, Dorothy M. "The Discipline of Nursing," *Nursing Outlook*, 26: 113–120, February, 1978.

Fagin, Claire M. "Primary Care as an Academic Discipline," *Nursing Outlook*, 26: 750–753, December, 1978.

Fenner, Kathleen. "Developing a Conceptual Framework," *Nursing Outlook*, 27: 122–126, February, 1979.

Hall, Kathryn V. "Current Trends in the Use of Conceptual Frameworks in Nursing Education," *Journal of Nursing Education*, 18: 26–29, April, 1979.

Johnson, Mauritz, "Definitions and Models in Curriculum Theory," in James Gress and David Purpel, eds., *Curriculum: An Introduction to the Field.* Berkeley, California: McCutchan Publishing Corporation, 1977, pp. 469–485.

Kelly, Jean. "The Philosophy as Part of the Total Curriculum Process," in *Faculty-Curriculum Development, Part IV: Curriculum Revision in Baccalaureate Nursing Education.* New York, National League for Nursing, Publication 15–1576, 1975.

Murdock, Jane E. "Regrouping for an Integrated Curriculum," *Nursing Outlook*, 26: 514–519, August, 1978.

National League for Nursing. Faculty-Curriculum Development, Part III: Conceptual Framework—Its Meaning and Function. New York: National League for Nursing, Publication 15–1558, 1975.

Partridge, Kay B. "Nursing Values in a Changing Society," *Nursing Outlook*, 26: 356–67, June, 1978.

Peterson, Carol J. "Questions Frequently Asked About the Development of a Conceptual Framework," *Journal of Nursing Education*, 16: 22–32, 1977.

Redman, Barbara K. "On Problems with Integrated Curricula in Nursing," *Journal of Nursing Education*, 17: 26–29, June, 1978.

Reilly, Dorothy E. *Behavioral Objectives in Nursing: Evaluation of Learner Attainment.* New York: Appleton-Century-Crofts, 1975.

———. "Why a Conceptual Framework?" *Nursing Outlook,* 23: 566–569, September, 1975.

Riehl, Joan P., and Roy, Sister Callista. *Conceptual Models for Nursing Practice.* New York: Appleton-Century-Crofts, 1974.

Roy, Sister Callista. "Adaptation: A Conceptual Framework for Nursing," *Nursing Outlook,* 18: 42–45, March, 1970.

Sullivan, Toni J. "An Experience with a Systems Approach to Curriculum Design," *Journal of Nursing Education,* 16: 25–34, March, 1977.

Treece, Eleanor Walters. "The Philosophical Basis of Nursing Education," *International Nursing Review,* 21: 13–20, 1974.

Williams, Carolyn. "The Nature and Development of Conceptual Frameworks," in Florence Downs and Juanita Fleming, eds., *Issues in Nursing Research.* New York: Appleton-Century-Crofts, 1979.

Yura, Helen. "Operationalizing the Philosophy, Conceptual Framework and Terminal Objectives," in *Curriculum Process for Developing or Revising a Baccalaureate Nursing Program.* New York, National League for Nursing, Publication 15-1700, 1978, pp. 35–46.

Chapter 3

Bloom, Benjamin, editor. *Taxonomy of Educational Objectives. Handbook I: Cognitive Domain.* New York: Longmans, Green and Co., 1956.

Bradford, Leland P., editor. *Human Forces in Teaching and Learning.* La Jolla, California: University Associates, Inc., 1976.

Conley, Virginia. *Curriculum and Instruction in Nursing.* Boston: Little, Brown and Co., 1973.

de Tornyay, Rheba. "Changing Student Relationships, Roles and Responsibilities," *Nursing Outlook,* 25: 188–193, March, 1977.

Gronlund, Norman E. *Stating Behavioral Objectives for Classroom Instruction.* New York: The Macmillan Co., 1970.

Harrow, Anita J. *Taxonomy of the Psychomotor Domain—A Guide for Developing Behavioral Objectives.* New York: David McKay, 1972.

Huckabay, Loucine M. *Conditions of Learning and Instruction in Nursing: Modularized.* St. Louis: C.V. Mosby Co., 1980.

Kapfer, Miriam B. *Behavioral Objectives in Curriculum Development.* Englewood Cliffs, New Jersey: Educational Technology Publications, 1971.

Krathwohl, David R., Bloom, Benjamin S., and Masia, Bertram B. *Taxonomy of Educational Objectives. Handbook II: Affective Domain.* New York: David McKay Co., Inc., 1956.

Mager, Robert F. *Preparing Instructional Objectives.* Belmont, California: Fearon Publishers, Inc., 1975.

Miller, Patricia. "Clinical Knowledge: A Needed Curriculum Emphasis," *Nursing Outlook,* 23: 222–224, April, 1975.

National League for Nursing. *Faculty-Curriculum Development, Part IV: Unifying the Curriculum—The Integrated Approach.* New York: National League for Nursing, Publication 15-1522, 1974.

Paduano, M. "Introducing Independent Study into the Nursing Curriculum," *Journal of Nursing Education,* 18: 34–37, April, 1979.

Pearson, Betty D. "Considerations of Student Clinical Assignments," *Journal of Nursing Education,* 16: 3–5, April, 1977.

Peterson, Carol Jean, Broderick, Mary E., Demarest, Lawrence, and Holey, Linda. *Competency-Based Curriculum and Instruction.* New York: National League for Nursing, 1979. Pub. No. 23-1770.

Pilette, Patricia. "Dewey Puts Behavioral Objectives into Perspective," *Journal of Nursing Education,* 15: 7–13, September, 1976.

Reilly, Dorothy. *Behavioral Objectives in Nursing: Evaluation of Learner Attainment.* New York: Appleton-Century-Crofts, 1975.

Sculco, Cynthia. "Development of a Taxonomy for the Nursing Process," *Journal of Nursing Education,* 17: 40–48, November, 1978.

Chapter 4

Apple, Michael W. "The Process and Ideology of Valuing in Educational Settings," in Arno Bellack and Herbert Kliebard, eds., *Curriculum and Evaluation.* Berkeley, California: McCutchan Publishing Co., 1977, pp. 468–493.

Bauman, Karen, and Kunka, Alice Kirkman. "Overhead Transparencies: The Overlooked Medium," *Nurse Educator,* 4: 21–25, July–August, 1979.

Chapman, Judy Jean. "Microteaching: How Students Learn Group Patient Education Skills," *Nurse Educator*, 3: 13–16, March–April, 1978.

Clark, Carolyn Chambers. *Classroom Skills for the Nurse Educator.* New York: Springer Publishing Co., 1978.

Coletta, Suzanne. "Values Clarification in Nursing: Why?" *American Journal of Nursing*, 78: 2057, December, 1978.

Conners, V. "Teaching Affective Behaviors," *Journal of Nursing Education*, 18: 33–39, June, 1979.

Corcoran, Sheila. "Should a Service Setting Be Used as a Learning Laboratory? An Ethical Question," *Nursing Outlook*, 25: 771–776, December, 1977.

Crancer, Joann, and Maury-Hess, Sharon. "Games: An Alternative to Pedagogical Instruction," *Journal of Nursing Education*, 19: 45–52, March, 1980.

de Tornyay, Rheba. *Strategies for Teaching Nursing.* New York: John Wiley and Sons, 1971.

Donaldson, Mary Louise. "Instructional Media as a Teaching Strategy," *Nurse Educator*, 4: 18–20, July–August, 1979.

Duane, Neil F. "An Audiovisual Overview," *Nurse Educator*, 4: 7–19, July–August, 1979.

Duley, John H. "Learning Through Field Experience," in *On College Teaching.* San Francisco: Jossey-Bass, Inc., 1978.

Eble, K. *The Craft of Teaching.* San Francisco: Jossey-Bass, Inc., 1977.

Flaskerud, Jacquelyn H. "Use of Vignettes to Elicit Responses Toward Broad Concepts," *Nursing Research*, 28: 210–212, July–August, 1979.

Flynn, John T., and Garber, Herbert, editors. *Assessing Behavior: Readings in Educational and Psychological Measurement.* Reading, Massachusetts: Addison-Wesley Publishing Co., 1967, pp. 316–328.

Guzzetta, Cathie E. "Relationship Between Stress and Learning," *Advances in Nursing Science,* 1: 35–49, July, 1979.

Hayter, Jean. "How Good Is the Lecture as a Teaching Method?" *Nursing Outlook,* 27: 274–277, April, 1979.

Hitchens, E.W. "Evaluation: The Graffiti Technique," *Journal of Nursing Education,* 18: 46–47, March, 1979.

Hogan, Rosemarie. "Making Clinical Assignments," *Nursing Outlook,* 24: 496–499, August, 1976.

Hogstel, Mildred D., and Ackley, Nancy L. "Making Team Teaching Work," *Nursing Outlook,* 27: 48–51, January, 1979.

Jeffers, J., and Christensen, M. "Using Simulation to Facilitate the Acquisition of Clinical Observational Skills," *Journal of Nursing Education,* 18: 29–32, June, 1979.

Jung, Steven M. "Application of the Critical Incident Technique in Developing Evaluative Measures," in David A. Payne, ed., *Curriculum Evaluation.* Lexington, Massachusetts: D.C. Heath and Co., 1974, pp. 207–210.

King, Elizabeth C. *Classroom Evaluation Strategies.* St. Louis: C.V. Mosby, Co., 1979.

Krawczyk, Rosemary. "Ethics: A Matter of Moral Development," *Nursing Outlook,* 78: 254–257, April, 1978.

Krumme, Ursel S. "The Case for Criterion-Referenced Measurement," *Nursing Outlook,* 23: 764–770, December, 1975.

Leininger, Madeleine. "Conflict and Conflict Resolution," *American Journal of Nursing,* 75: 292–296, February, 1975.

Malasanos, Lois, and Tichy, Anna Marie. "The Bedside Clinic-Nursing Rounds as a Teaching Strategy," *Journal of Nursing Education,* 16: 10–15, June, 1977.

Marriner, Ann. "Student Self-Evaluation and the Contracted Grade," *Nursing Forum,* 13: 131–135, 1974.

McGoran, S. "Teaching Students Self-Awareness," *American Journal of Nursing*, 78: 859–61, May, 1978.

McGrane, Helen F. "Tape Recorded Evaluation: A Method of Teaching," *Journal of Nursing Education*, 14: 10–17, January, 1975.

McGuire, Christine H., Solomon, Lawrence M., and Bashook, Philip G. *Construction and Use of Written Simulations.* New York: The Psychological Corporation, 1976.

Page, Gordon G., and Saunders, Peggy. "Written Simulation in Nursing," *Journal of Nursing Education*, 17: 28–32, April, 1978.

Payne, David A. *The Assessment of Learning: Cognitive and Affective.* Lexington, Massachusetts: D.C. Heath and Co., 1974.

Pearson, Betty D. "A Model for Clinical Evaluation," *Nursing Outlook*, 23: 232–235, April, 1975.

Perry, S. "Teaching Strategy and Learner Performance," *Journal of Nursing Education*, 18: 25–27, January, 1979.

Popham, W. James. *Educational Evaluation.* Englewood Cliffs, New Jersey: Prentice-Hall, Inc., 1975.

Reilly, Dorothy E. *Behavioral Objectives in Nursing: Evaluation of Learner Attainment.* New York: Appleton-Century-Crofts, 1975.

———. editor. *Teaching and Evaluating the Affective Domain in Nursing.* New York: Charles B. Slack, Inc., 1978.

Schmalenberg, Claudia. "Making and Using Slides," *Nurse Educator*, 4: 12–15, July–August, 1979.

Schweer, J., and Gebbie, K. *Creative Teaching in Clinical Nursing*, 3rd ed., St. Louis: C.V. Mosby Co., 1976.

Smith, D. "The Effect of Values on Clinical Teaching," in Janet Williamson, ed., *Current Perspectives in Nursing Education: The Changing Scene.* St. Louis: C.V. Mosby Co., 1976.

Smoyak, Shirley A. "Teaching as Coaching," *Nursing Outlook*, 26: 361–366, June, 1978.

Uustal, Diane. "Values Clarification in Nursing: Application to Practice," *American Journal of Nursing*, 78: 2058–2063, December, 1978.

Voight, J. "Assessing Clinical Performance: A Model for Competency," *Journal of Nursing Education*, 18: 30–33, April, 1979.

Watkins, Carolyn. "Student Evaluation by Computer," *Nursing Outlook*, 23: 449–452, July, 1975.

Williamson, Janet, and Therrien, Barbara. "The Nurse Preceptor," in Janet Williamson, ed., *Current Perspectives in Nursing Education*, Vol II, St. Louis: C.V. Mosby Co., 1978.

Yeaw, E. "Problem Solving as a Method of Teaching Strategies in Classroom and Clinical Teaching," *Journal of Nursing Education*, 18: 16–22, September, 1979.

Chapter 5

Bellack, Arno A., and Kliebard, Herbert M., editors. *Curriculum and Evaluation*. Berkeley, California: McCutchan Publishing Corporation, 1977.

Benner, R., and Benner, P. "Follow-through Evaluation: A Resource for Curriculum Planning and Development," *Nurse Educator*, 4: 16–21, September–October, 1979.

Gordon, Marjory, and Anello, Michael. "A Systematic Approach to Curriculum Revision," *Nursing Outlook*, 22: 306–309, May, 1974.

Green, Joan L., and Stone, James C. *Curriculum Evaluation: Theory and Practice*. New York: Springer Publishing Co., 1977.

Hamilton, Arthur S., and others, editors. *Beyond the Numbers Game: A Reader in Educational Evaluation.* Berkeley, California: McCutchan Publishing Corporation. 1977.

LaBelle, Beverly M., and Egan, Ellen C. "Follow-Up Studies in Nursing: A Case for Determining Whether Program Objectives Are Achieved," *Journal of Nursing Education,* 14: 7–13, August, 1975.

Lee, Lettie. "An Investigation of the Effects of Clinical Experience on Cognitive Gains," *Journal of Nursing Education,* 18: 27–37, September, 1979.

Lynch, Eleanor A., Torres, Gertrude, and Yura, Helen. *Faculty-Curriculum Development, Part II, Curriculum Evaluation.* New York: National League for Nursing, Publication 15–1530, 1974.

Meleis, Afaf I., and Benner, Patricia. "Process or Product Evaluation?" *Nursing Outlook,* 23: 303–307, May, 1975.

National League for Nursing. *Program Evaluation.* New York: National League for Nursing, Publication 15–1738, 1978.

Weinstein, E. Brown, and Wahlstrom, M.W. "Characteristics of the Successful Nursing Student," *Journal of Nursing Education,* 19: 53–59, March, 1980.

Chapter 6

Torres, Gertrude. "Curriculum Process—Problems and Concerns," in *Faculty-Curriculum Development, Part I: The Process of Curriculum Development.* New York: National League for Nursing, Publication 15–1521, 1974, pp. 9–13.

Chapter 7

Coffey, Lou. *Modules for Independent-Individual Learning in Nursing.* Philadelphia: F.A. Davis Co., 1975.

del Bueno, Dorothy. "Competency Based Education," *Nurse Educator,* 3: 10-14, May-June, 1978.

Duley, John H. "Learning Through Field Experience," *On College Teaching.* San Francisco: Jossey-Bass, Inc., 1978.

Gengiades, W., and others. *New Schools for a New Age.* Santa Monica: Goodyear Publishing Co., 1977.

Knapp, Joan, and Sharon, Amiel. *A Compendium of Assessment Techniques.* Princeton, New Jersey: Cooperative Assessment of Experiential Learning, Educational Testing Service, 1975.

Knowles, M. *The Adult Learner: A Neglected Species.* Houston: Gulf Publishing Co., 1973.

Malarkey, Louise. "The Older Student—Stress or Success on Campus," *Journal of Nursing Education,* 18: 15-19, February, 1979.

Milton, Ohmer. *Alternatives to the Traditional.* San Francisco: Jossey-Bass, Inc., 1972.

Notter, Lucille E., and Robey, Marguerite. *The Open Curriculum in Nursing Education.* New York: National League for Nursing, Publication 19-1799, 1979.

Rogers, Suzanne. "Testing the RN Student's Skills," *Nursing Outlook,* 24: 446-449, July, 1976.

Willingham, Warren W. *Principles of Good Practice in Assessing Experiential Learning.* Columbia, Maryland: Cooperative Assessment of Experiential Learning, 1977.

Index

NLN Achievement tests, 91, 93
Norm-referenced evaluation, 91
Nursing:
conceptualizing, 32–34, 36
medical *vs.* integrated model, 75–79
as a process, 15–16, 54
in sample curriculum, 113–115 *tab.*,
119, 127–129 *tab.*, 138
Nursing courses:
balancing with other courses, 21, 58–60
credit-by-examination, 163
in sample curriculum, 131–35 *tab.*,
136, 139–41 *tab.*
and sequencing of content, 41

O

Organizational structure, 5–7
Output component, 26, 102, 105–6, 173

P

Parallel design, 56 *fig.* 57
implications for transfer students, 160
Parent institution:
degree limits, 58
goals of, 32
impact on curriculum development,
8–9
resources, 55
Philosophy:
and beliefs, 30
and concepts, 30–31
defined, 29–30
and propositions, 31
and theory, 31 (*See also* Curriculum
philosophy)
Prerequisites:
and credit-by-examination, 163
in curriculum design, 22, 59
implications for transfer students, 160,
163
in sample curriculum, 130, 131–33
tab.
and sequencing of content, 41
Pretesting, 104
Prioritization:
in course outline, 66–67
in directive stage, 19
Process:
and characteristics of graduate, 48
as content, 117
defined, 16, 173
distinguished from content, 4–5
and level and course objectives, 60, 63

Process (cont.)
nursing as, 15–16, 54, 119, 138 (*See
also* Horizontal strands)
Progressive design, 56 *fig.*, 57, 80
Propositions:
defined, 31, 173
developing, 36–37
effect on transfer student policies, 157
as guidelines to curriculum design, 55,
57–58
from sample curriculum, 112, 116 *tab.*,
122–24 *tab.*
validating, 37–38

R

Research:
in directive stage, 19
in sample curriculum, 119
Responsibility:
of faculty, 3–5, 10
in sample curriculum, 120
Role development, in sample curriculum,
120

S

Science requirements:
credit-by-examination, 163
in curriculum design, 55, 59
in sample curriculum, 134–35 *tab.*,
136
Semimedical model, 76–79, 173
Sequencing of content:
in content map, 63
and course outline, 67
design guidelines, 55
implications for transfer students, 160
and motivation, 80
of prerequisites, 59
rationale, 68 *tab.*
theoretical framework, 41–42 (*See also*
Content)
Simulation tests, 95 *tab.*
Skills:
in sample curriculum, 115 *tab.*
teaching methods, 84
theoretical base, 41
Small group activities, 87 *tab.*
Society:
concept in sample curriculum, 113–15
tab., 119, 125 *tab.*, 137–38
meaning of term, 39
Specialities, 75, 76 (*See also* Medical
model)